Pulmonary Rehabilitation

Pulmonary Rehabilitation
From Hospital to Home

Jerry A. O'Ryan, A.A.S., B.S., C.R.T.T., R.R.T.
Center Manager, Travenol Home Respiratory Therapy
Cincinnati and Dayton, Ohio
Former Chief Therapist, Pulmonary Rehabilitation
Grandview and Southview Hospitals
Dayton, Ohio

Donald G. Burns, D.O., F.A.C.O.I., F.C.C.P.
Clinical Professor of Medicine (Pulmonary)
Ohio University, Athens, Ohio
Chairman, Department of Pulmonology
Director, Respiratory Therapy
Grandview and Southview Hospitals
Dayton, Ohio

YEAR BOOK MEDICAL PUBLISHERS, INC.
CHICAGO

Reprinted, July 1984

Library of Congress Cataloging in Publication Data

O'Ryan, Jerry.
   Pulmonary rehabilitation.

   Bibliography: p.
   Includes index.
   1. Respiratory therapy.   2. Lungs—Diseases—Patients
—Rehabilitation.   I. Burns, Donald G.   II. Title.
[DNLM: 1. Lung diseases—Rehabilitation.   WF 600 P9865]
RM161.079   1984   615.8'36   84-2198
ISBN 0-8151-6550-1

Sponsoring editor: Diana L. McAninch
Production project manager: Dorothy J. Mulligan
Editing supervisor: Frances M. Perveiler
Copyeditor: Kareen Snider
Proofroom supervisor: Shirley E. Taylor

To Nancy, my ultimate zenith

J.A.O.'R.

Contributors

Tali A. Conine, R.P.T., D.H.S.
University of British Columbia
Faculty of Medicine
School of Rehabilitation Medicine
Vancouver, British Columbia, Canada

Jerome E. Holliday, Ph.D.
Director of Pulmonary Biofeedback
St. Louis University Hospital
St. Louis, Missouri

Jeff Lucas, R.R.T.
Clinical Specialist
T & M Oxygen
Cleveland, Ohio

Jack K. Plummer, Ph.D.
Director, Division of Psychology
Gaylord Hospital
Wallingford, Connecticut

Contents

Foreword xiii
Preface xv
Acknowledgments xix

1. Introduction 1

2. The Selection of the Pulmonary Rehabilitation Candidate . . . 5
   What Is Fitness for the COLD Patient? 6
   Evaluating Objective Gains 8
   Evaluating Subjective Gains 10
   Summary. 15

3. Pathophysiology of Chronic and Acute Lung Disease. 17
   Asthma 17
   Emphysema 21
   Chronic Bronchitis. 23
   Fatigue of the Diaphragm 24
   Pulmonary Rehabilitation Considerations 27
   Summary. 29

4. Diagnostic Techniques for Assessing Pulmonary Dysfunction . . 32
   History 32
   Physical Examination 34
   Laboratory Data. 34
   Chest X-ray. 35
   Pulmonary Function Studies 36
   Pulmonary Exercise Studies. 37
   Physiologic Picture of the Patient 43
   Summary. 44

5. Hands-on Evaluation 46
   The Patient Interview 46
   Review of Systems. 49
   Physical Examination 50
   Summary. 63

ix

6. **Pulmonary Rehabilitation Techniques** **64**
   Principles of Breathing Training and Exercise 64
   Breathing Training Techniques 66
   Principles of Exercise 71
   Techniques of Exercise. 72
   Writing the Exercise Prescription 78
   Summary. 81

7. **Biofeedback** **85**
   Review of the Literature 86
   Anxiety and the COLD Patient 89
   Breathing Retraining With Biofeedback. 102
   Professional Qualifications for Performing Pulmonary
   Biofeedback 109

8. **Oxygen Therapy** **112**
   Normal Pulmonary Vascular Anatomy and Physiology. 112
   Pulmonary Hypertension. 115
   Patient Selection for Oxygen Therapy 118
   Objectives of Oxygen Therapy. 119
   Oxygen Delivery Systems 121
   Summary. 132

9. **Nutrition**. **135**
   Metabolic Changes 135
   Physiology 136
   Nutritional Assessment. 140
   Initial Assessment 141
   Nutritional Therapy 141
   Summary. 144

10. **Psychosocial Factors in Pulmonary Rehabilitation** **146**
    A Paradigm of Pulmonary Rehabilitation 153
    The Multidisciplinary Team Approach 153
    Self-Help Groups 155
    Death and Dying: Patients' Rights 157
    Treatment of the Whole Person 159
    Behavioral Techniques 160
    Sexuality and Disability 162
    Summary. 166

11. **Patient Education** **173**
    The Objectives of Patient Education 173
    Motivation to Learn 175
    Best Way to Teach 176

Teaching the Young Learner 177
Evaluation of Patient Education 177
Teaching Patients: A Helping Relationship 178
Summary. 180

12. **Starting a Pulmonary Rehabilitation Program.** **182**
The First Step: Marketing 182
The Multidisciplinary Approach 185
Obtaining Personnel 189
Where and When Is Pulmonary Rehabilitation Performed? . . 190
Phase I-IV Concept 191
Charting and Reporting Systems. 191
Equipment 192
Departmental Layout 193
Summary. 196

13. **Home Care.** **199**
The Role of the Home-Care Team 199
The Patient and Family's Responsibilities 201
Requirements for Safe Home Care. 203
Cost of Home Care 206
An Alternative to Hospital-Based Home Care 208
Summary. 209

14. **Home Ventilator Care** **211**
Identifying the Prime Candidate for Home Mechanical
Ventilation 212
Home-Care Team Members 213
Primary Care Givers: The Family 216
Clinical Profile of Ideal Home Ventilator Patient. 217
Cost Considerations 217
Evaluation of the Home 218
Instructional Routine. 220
Ancillary Equipment Selection 222
Ventilator Selection 223
Equipment Decontamination and Infection Control 227
Community Services. 229
Follow-Up and Continuing Care. 230
Summary. 232

15. **Audiovisuals and Print Media; Aids and Organizations** **234**
Audiovisual Aids 234
Pamphlets and Brochures. 238
Organizations 239

Contents

Appendix A **241**
    Calculating Relative Fractions of Inspired Oxygen (FI_{O2}) . . . 241

Apendix B **243**
    High-Calorie, High-Protein Sample Menu 243
    High Protein, Weight-Reduction Sample Menu 244
    Notes 244

Index **247**

Foreword

PULMONARY REHABILITATION is an established method of care for patients with advanced chronic productive pulmonary disease which has altered the lives of hundreds of thousands of people who suffer from emphysema. What is pulmonary rehabilitation? It is a form of individually tailored treatment strategies that include patient and family education, breathing training, breathing exercises, physical reconditioning and in selective cases, home oxygen. In addition, pulmonary rehabilitation requires attention to good nutrition, positive health habits, and a new outlook on life designed to enhance the happiness of the individual.

It is true that emphysema is characterized by premature morbidity and mortality. All evidence points to the fact that rehabilitative techniques forestall both morbidity and mortality. There is more to life than just surviving, however, and experts in the field of respiratory care and pulmonary medicine have been interested in improving the quality of life. Pulmonary rehabilitation probably does more to improve life quality than anything else and it certainly does so by keeping patients active and living at home rather than in hospitals or extended care facilities.

New technology such as home oxygen equipment has greatly added to our armamentarium for home care. Today, hundreds of thousands of patients can reap the benefits of oxygen in their own home and they can also be active using portable devices. But oxygen is not for everyone. It is reserved for those who have certain consequences of emphysema resulting in marked loss of oxygen and associated physical impairments, including cor pulmonale.

This book is written by experts who have participated in all aspects of rehabilitative care for many years. A wealth of material is contained that will interest both members of the profession, i.e., physicians, respiratory therapists and nurses, as well as the patients and their families this team aims to serve. Many of the excellent illustrations will offer new insights into methods of care and specific techniques that may be valuable for many patients.

As one who has been highly interested in the subject of this book, I commend the authors and particularly Jerry O'Ryan who organized and edited this important book. Through their efforts, more physicians, respiratory therapists and nurses will get involved in pulmonary rehabilitation because of the value it offers to patients and their families.

THOMAS L. PETTY, M.D.
PROFESSOR OF MEDICINE
DIRECTOR, WEBB-WARING LUNG INSTITUTE
CO-HEAD, DIVISION OF PULMONARY SCIENCES
DENVER, COLORADO

Preface

PULMONARY REHABILITATION (and its domiciliary neighbor, home care) are currently where pulmonary function and diagnostic techniques were ten years ago, and where pediatric respiratory therapy/neonatology was perhaps six years ago. Both of these fields are now relatively firmly established. In contrast, pulmonary rehabilitation is right at that threshold. One may think of pulmonary rehabilitation as respiratory care's new frontier. It is for this reason that this book has been written.

This author's experience with pulmonary rehabilitation in all its forms has shown that practically "everyone" is doing rehabilitative work with chronic and acute lung-diseased patients. A closer look reveals that "everyone," however, is doing it in vast and varying degrees, and very few are applying all its principles and techniques. Indeed, even fewer are aware of the total spectrum available to the practitioner and his patient. It is for these reasons, too, that this book has been written.

Empirically and scientifically, pulmonary rehabilitation is midpoint in the "discovery" stage. Although some research results and applications of those findings are being used in the clinical setting, practitioners (i.e., physicians, respiratory therapists, nurses, and all other health and related professionals dealing with the chronic lung-diseased patient) will find pulmonary rehabilitation a new frontier for further research, new methodologies, and clinical innovations.

A working definition constructed in 1974 by the American College of Chest Physicians' Committee on Pulmonary Rehabilitation defined pulmonary rehabilitation as follows:

An art of medical practice wherein an individually tailored multidisciplinary program is formulated which, through accurate diagnosis, therapy, emotional support, and education stabilizes or reverses both the physio- and the psychopathology of pulmonary disease and attempts to return the patient to the highest possible functional capacity allowed by his pulmonary handicap and overall life situation.

This book is intended for anyone dealing with chronic or acute lung-diseased patients whose lives have benefited from the science *and* art of pulmonary rehabilitative techniques. This would include respiratory therapists and pulmonary physician specialists, but it would also extend to nurses, physical therapists, occupational therapists, cardiopulmonary technologists, and dietitians. Those involved with the patient's hospital-to-home transition, i.e., discharge planners and social service workers, should also find much of this book invaluable and insightful. All of these may be thought of as the "hospital-based" professionals dealing with the chronic lung-diseased patient. Those professions that are "community centered" include the home health agencies, hospice workers, and durable medical equipment dealers. All three play a central role for the patient desiring to return to his domicile for convalescence in familiar surroundings. The last half of chapter 7 and all of chapters 13 and 14 were written for those dealing with the home-care aspects of the pulmonary patient.

Third-party payers are encouraged to peruse this book, especially those chapters pertaining to oxygen therapy and home care. It is ironic that the insurance reimbursement system, which pays for high-quality intensive care for the ventilator-bound patient, could have saved tenfold by renumerating for prophylactic care, i.e., pulmonary rehabilitation, prior to the insidious exacerbations leading to the patient's repeated hospital admissions.

It is also suggested that those with legislative involvement scrutinize these pages, because at this writing (and perhaps for quite a time to come), legislators have not been convinced of the merits of preventative health care and long-term treatment of the chronically ill.

Last, but not least, students will not only find this book academically informative, but it may lead them to consider this area of pulmonary medicine as their chosen specialty.

Costs for pulmonary rehabilitation are virtually always less than hospitalization. More important, studies have shown that the maintenance-type care that outpatient pulmonary rehabilitation provides not only decreases any future hospital admissions the patient may require, but also decreases total hospital days per readmission.

Because pulmonary rehabilitation programs derive from many conventional respiratory therapy and related pulmonary care modalities and diagnostic techniques, hospitals should find the upstart costs of initiating a conscientious, well-thought-out program a minimal expenditure. The medically necessary ancillary laboratory, radiologic, pulmonary diagnostic, and other required testing usually should more than offset any negative operating costs of a pulmonary rehabilitation program.

Finally, it is for the above reasons along with their ramifications that this book should be read. We will soon see pulmonary rehabilitation take its place alongside pulmonary diagnostics and pediatric/neonatal respiratory care as another firmly-established specialty of the respiratory practitioner.

Just as the scope and level of medical practice varies throughout the health care field, so does the level and resultant practice of pulmonary rehabilitation. One of the objectives of this book, both in philosophy and practice, is to provide a point of reference for the present and future practice of this new subdiscipline. Ben Franklin said, "Each man's" does not go alike, yet each believes his own." Ben was referring to a man's timepiece, but the analogy is perfect here. I trust our work will help the reader to attain a more congruent practice of this most exciting new frontier called pulmonary rehabilitation.

JERRY A. O'RYAN

Acknowledgments

THIS WORK COULD NOT have come to fruition without the assistance of many people. As a reader (and now as a writer) I often peruse the preluding pages of a book to see what ancillary assistance, in body and spirit, has been offered the author. I often see glowing praise of those mentioned in the obligatory acknowledgments section. I now know why. Writing can be an almost impossible task, a significant time-consuming task to be sure. That arduous task is made significantly easier by the physical and moral support of others.

It has been said that writing is easy: "You merely open your veins and bleed." It has also been noted that "writing is merely rewriting what you've already rewritten." Although I agree 100% with these keen observations, I would like to add a third, and possibly more pragmatic, experienced-based outlook. My advice is as follows: Surround yourself with the best possible people to help you, listen to them carefully, and allow their fresh ideas to renew your literary endeavors. The following people, in many and various ways, have performed just that task for me.

It is, of course, imperative that I begin by acknowledging the five people who provided 50% of the pages of this work, my coauthors. Since they are formally introduced to the reader on the title page, and proof of their writing talents is contained within this book, I can only personally say a deep-felt "thank you" to Donald G. Burns, D.O., Jerome E. Holliday, Ph.D., Jack K. Plummer, Ph.D., Jeff Lucas, R.R.T., and Tali A. Conine, D.H.S., R.P.T.

Because of my reviewers and their words of wisdom, wit, criticism, and encouragement, my job was made much easier. I am truly flattered and grateful to Thomas L. Petty, M.D., who took time from his busy schedule to write an excellent critique and personal words of a morale-boosting nature. Dr. Petty's foreword to this book multiplies a debt I am honored to owe. Robert J. MacDonell, M.A., R.R.T., staff development coordinator at Harper Grace Hospitals in Detroit, wrote one of the most extensive (and most appreciated) critiques of my manuscript. Thank you, Bob; your important comments only made me look that much better when I interpolated them into the final work. Stan Gloss, R.R.T., assistant professor of respiratory therapy at Quinnipiac College in Hamden, Conn. gave much wise, constructive criticism and support during the intermediary stages of my writing. His suggestions greatly assisted me in my final drafts.

There is one significant person who helped round out this book *and* its editor. Karla Snavely, R.R.T., pulmonary rehabilitation coordinator at Grandview and Southview Hospitals in Dayton, Ohio, lent her film-review talents in chapter 15. Karla also compiled the list of professional organizations in that chapter. More importantly, she tolerated my sometimes erratic behavior and shared my sense of the incredulous over many things for many months. Thanks, "Libby."

Four other persons and one group also contributed directly to the work. Dale Borts, R.R.T., inservice educator for respiratory therapy at Grandview and Southview Hospitals, took many of the photographs for this book. Essentially, Dale was an artistic photographer turned technical photographer, and he rapidly became good at it. Dale's photographs are all those in the book, except as noted otherwise by credit line. Linda Mullen patiently executed the line drawings in Chapters 6 and 10. Linda's excellent illustrations complement the author's words. David K. Wildasin, R.R.T., supervisor, inpatient care, Southview Hospital, kindly wrote Appendix A: Calculating Relative Fractions of Inspired Oxygen. Dave Baker, R.R.T., special procedures coordinator at Grandview and Southview Hospitals, researched and wrote the exercise prescription information in Chapter 6. Finally, four dietitians from Grandview Hospital wrote the sample menu items in Appendix B. They are Rebecca Barnett, R.D., Holly Channell, R.D., Pamela Cleveland, R.D., and Kitty McHugh, R.D.

A very special thanks is warmly extended to Kathy Murray, C.R.T.T., pulmonary rehabilitation staff therapist at Grandview and Southview Hospitals, for her excellent typing of original drafts of the manuscript.

Carol Grove made my primary contributing author's (Dr. Donald G. Burns) work on this book much easier. Thank you, Carol, for helping my esteemed writing colleague meet his deadlines. Thanks to Denise Vincent for typing one cold rainy day in March 1983. Thanks to Geoffrey Sleeper, R.R.T., for his special assistance to Jeff Lucas, R.R.T., in Chapter 14. Thank you, Loma Pallman and Candy Winteregg, librarians at Grandview Hospital, for your literature searches and other various and sundry tasks you performed for me for 2½ years.

This book would not have been possible without the coordinating talents of my medical editor at Year Book, Diana McAninch. Not only did Diana do the job for which her employer hired her (and did it well), she also patiently listened to me over the phone many times these past 28 months.

I confer upon Fran Perveiler, editing supervisor at Year Book, and her staff an honorary combined respiratory therapy/medical degree. Fran and her group's copyediting talents made the final manuscript the perfected piece that we believe it to be.

Two final acknowledgments are in order, and these mark the beginning, as well as a most important intermediate point, respectively, in my professional career and life.

Thank you Robert A. Dittmar, R.R.T. #26, for having faith to hire me for my very first "inhalation" therapy job on October 17, 1967.

Finally, thanks to Gail Sheehy, author of *Passages* and *Pathfinders*. My wife, Nancy, brought home the latter book to me in March of this year, at a time when this source of inspiration and guidance was sorely needed.

JERRY A. O'RYAN
Thanksgiving Day, 1983

1 / Introduction

JERRY A. O'RYAN, B.S., R.R.T.

AS OF THIS WRITING, chronic respiratory diseases are the third leading cause of death in the United States, determining about one in ten deaths among our citizens. In contrast to this surge in respiratory disease and related deaths has been the significant decline in cardiovascular disease mortality, down by 24% during 1968 to 1978.

Respiratory-related problems are implicated in 20% of all physician contacts and in 12% of short-term hospitalizations. An estimate of the direct and indirect costs of these illnesses is about $45 billion annually. There are more lost work days (31.3 million annual person-days) than from any other category of illness. Respiratory illnesses rank sixth among conditions leading to early retirement due to disability (statistics from the American Lung Association (ALA) and the American Thoracic Society (ATS) May 1982: "Report and Recommendations of the Task Force on Federal Lung Research").

Often, emphasis on treatment of respiratory illnesses, including the main disease subject of this book, chronic obstructive lung ailments, has been after-the-fact. This is to say that often more time and effort, albeit in good faith, is put into treating the patient's condition after he has reached an exacerbative level or acute stage. Perhaps both parties in the health care schema are partially to blame for this tardy approach: (1) the health care professional, for failing to treat the problem in its very early onset and (2) the patient, for failing to bring the insidious (but subjectively obvious) symptoms to his health care professional. The patient may also be held liable for a second misdemeanor — that of harboring bad health habits, especially tobacco smoking.

Nevertheless, once the disease is noted, it should be aggressively evaluated and treated. Since "preventative" care is the health care model for today, hopefully both of the above-mentioned parties will attend to the problem before a minor symptom becomes pluralistic and the whole syndrome pattern develops, i.e., coughing, wheezing, severe dyspnea, decreased expiration flows, cor pulmonale, etc.

The process by which one may at least partially if not greatly decrease the above problems is called *pulmonary rehabilitation*. While pulmonary

1

rehabilitation is not a panacea, it can certainly go a long way to restore some semblance of normality to the chronic obstructive lung-diseased (COLD) patient's daily lifestyle, as delineated by the American College of Chest Physicians in the preface of this book.

Much thought and thousands of man-hours went into the preparation of this book. "Find the need and endeavor to meet it" is a quote from Dale Sinclair, the founder of one of the largest community colleges in the United States, Sinclair Community College in Dayton, Ohio. There was indeed a need to meet in the writing of this book on pulmonary rehabilitation. The editor and contributing authors did not wish to compile a cookbook-type publication; at the same time, they wanted the book to serve those at the entry phase of pulmonary rehabilitation. On the other hand, they desired to also serve an eclectic group of those at various stages in pulmonary rehabilitation programs. We believe the above criteria have been fairly well met.

The authors have purposely left out areas of general information that can be easily obtained from a plethora of other books and publications on this subject. For example, standard respiratory therapy modalities such as intermittent positive-pressure breathing (IPPB), aerosol, chest physical therapy, and updraft medication delivery devices are not reiterated.

New material that has not been traditionally related to the field of respiratory therapy is found in Chapters 7, 8, 9, and 10. This material, much of which in the editor's opinion is unprecedented, may even prove beneficial to areas outside the field of pulmonary rehabilitation. If so, then those respective authors (Holliday, Burns, Plummer, and Conine) will have produced material with a more far-reaching effect than what the editor required (so much the better).

The following briefly outlines the contents of this first edition; the thought that went into its preparation and the therapeutic philosophy it seeks to evoke will hopefully be apparent after a complete reading of the work.

Chapter 2, "Selection of the Pulmonary Rehabilitation Candidate," is a natural starting point for this book. This chapter compares the COLD patient with the healthy individual, redefining the concept of physical fitness for the pulmonary-impaired person. The reader is advised at the beginning of the book how to evaluate *objective* and *subjective* gains made by the patient in a pulmonary rehabilitation program.

Chapter 3, "Pathophysiology of Chronic and Acute Lung Disease," reviews the basic tenets of the three common types of pulmonary problems: asthma, emphysema, and chronic bronchitis. It concludes with the book's first suggestions for pulmonary rehabilitative techniques.

Chapter 4, "Diagnostic Techniques for Assessing Pulmonary Dysfunction," is an excellent laboratory summary of suggested testing profiles needed for an objective assay of the patient's pulmonary status. Starting with the time-honored history taking and pulmonary function test, the chapter lists various exercise studies such as the 12-minute walking test and instructs the reader how to assess the data.

Chapter 5, "Hands-on Evaluation," is a most pragmatic chapter and should prove to be especially useful to respiratory therapists, medical students, nurse clinicians, physician's assistants, and others interested in performing a comprehensive bedside or office respiratory assessment.

Chapter 6, "Pulmonary Rehabilitation Techniques," presents some of the most important information in the book, including the principles and application of the actual breathing training and exercise modalities for the patient. Diaphragmatic pursed-lip breathing, range-of-motion exercises, walking, treadmill, and cycling are discussed with their various merits and limits addressed. A new therapeutic modality, *inspiratory muscle training*, makes its first debut in a nonperiodical publication. Many illustrations and tables supplement the material in this chapter.

Chapter 7, "Biofeedback for Pulmonary Rehabilitation," is the first hardbound treatment of this subject. The author explains this relaxation technique, which uses light, sound, and other self-regulated external devices to help the COLD patient achieve qualitatively and quantitatively beneficial breathing patterns. Many tables, illustrations, and photographs augment this chapter.

Chapter 8, "Oxygen Therapy," is a review of normal anatomy and physiology of the arteriolar-capillary-venule system as well as an explanation of pulmonary hypertension as a precursor of the patient's requirement for long-term oxygen therapy. The ATS oxygen usage guidelines suggest optimal oxygen dosage levels. Staying with the concept of rehabilitative oxygen needs for ambulating and bed-bound patients, the various oxygen systems (gaseous, liquid, and concentrator) are discussed. Benefits and limitations of each are addressed through the text, tables, figures, and photographs.

Chapter 9, "Nutrition," explains the metabolic changes occurring as a result of chronic lung disease. The author shows how the daily caloric requirement is related to the patient's oxygen requirements as determined by oxygen consumption. Nutritional assessment and nutritional therapy are explained.

Chapter 10, "Psychosocial Aspects of Pulmonary Rehabilitation," is a detailed treatment of the subject with over 100 references. The concept of the multidisciplinary team approach, self-help groups, and patients' rights are discussed as well as sexuality and disability as they relate to the pulmonary rehabilitation patient.

Chapter 11, "Patient Education," offers pragmatic, educational tips on understanding the COLD patient and teaching to his level of understanding. The three conventional teaching methods (cognitive, affective, and psychomotor) are discussed in relation to the health care teaching environment. Teaching is defined as a "helping relationship," and the reader is advised to approach patient education with this concept in mind.

Chapter 12, "Starting a Pulmonary Rehabilitation Program," informs the reader how to begin, market, and perpetuate a pulmonary rehabilitation program regardless of scope or physical size of the department. It may be desirable to read this chapter prior to reading chapter 2. Reporting forms and other samples of paperwork are illustrated in this section. In this chapter, the individual roles of the multidisciplinary team members are delineated from the patient's perspective.

Chapter 13, "Home Care," instructs the reader in extending the pulmonary rehabilitation process into the patient's domicile. A comprehensive discussion of the two key home-care health providers, the respiratory therapist and nurse, is given. Guidelines for the selection of home-care equipment and monitoring in-home therapy are provided and the patient's and family members' duties and responsibilities delineated. Finally, a discussion of home-care costs is given with comparisons to hospital costs. The advantages and disadvantages of having hospital-based respiratory therapists provide home care are explored.

Chapter 14, "Home Ventilator Care," serves as follow-up to Chapter 13 as one viable alternative to a specific long-term problem occurring in the hospital, that of prolonged ventilatory support for the otherwise physiologically stable patient, The author proceeds through the entire hospital-to-home transition of long-term ventilatory support. Each home-care step is discussed with many helpful hints to make for a smooth transition to the home. Many tables, figures, and photographs are used to explain and illustrate the concept of ventilator care in the home setting.

Chapter 15, "Audiovisuals and Print Media; Aids and Organizations," serves as a compendium of tapes, films, literature, and places to write for additional information. Three audiovisual films dealing with chronic lung disease are reviewed. Addresses of most professional organizations that may have additional information related to pulmonary rehabilitation or pulmonary ailments are provided for the reader's convenience.

Finally, appendices conclude the book. Appendix A shows the reader how to calculate relative fractions of inspired oxygen and is meant as a companion to Chapter 8, "Oxygen Therapy." Appendix B provides an example of a high-calorie, high-protein menu and is intended as a companion piece to Chapter 9, "Nutrition."

2 / The Selection of the Pulmonary Rehabilitation Candidate

JERRY A. O'RYAN, B.S., R.R.T.

THE INTENT OF THIS CHAPTER is to set the general premise for the selection of pulmonary rehabilitation candidates by examining the rationale behind the selection process. Some patients make good candidates for entry into the pulmonary rehabilitation process. Some do not. While even the novice practitioner would realize that the end-stage terminally ill patient would not be considered a candidate, there are, unfortunately, patients at the other end of the spectrum who also may not be viable candidates. For the latter an example would be the extremely noncompliant patient who may be physiologically salvageable, but lacks either the interest or long-term commitment to the regimen of a comprehensive pulmonary rehabilitation program.

There are gray areas at both ends of the spectrum. It is not the intent of this chapter to examine every microcosm of the selection process; however, a fairly comprehensive profile of the viable candidate can be gained by the reader through this chapter's definition of *physical fitness* and what it means for the chronic obstructive lung-diseased (COLD) patient. Equally important is the chapter's examination of the *objective* and *subjective* gains the patient is wholly or partially expected to obtain as a result of his participation in a pulmonary rehabilitation program.

This introductory chapter will also look at the measuring, monitoring, and evaluation procedures that allow some meaningful insight into the individual patient's progress and that provide part of the basis for the acceptance of the individual patient into a comprehensive pulmonary rehabilitation program. This is not to say that the volumes of past, present, and future investigators' reports based on group studies have no clinical application. Indeed, this book is largely based upon such studies, as evidenced by the references. However, the intent of this chapter is to focus on the individual patient by providing the premise for the various pathologic assessment, clinical diagnostic, and eventual prescribing mechanisms discussed in Chapters 3, 4, and 5. The reader can then use that information to evaluate the results of the patient's endeavors at breathing training and exercise as discussed in Chapter 6. This chapter will also apprise the reader of the science and philosophy reflected in the practice of pulmonary rehabilitation.

What Is Fitness For The COLD Patient?

In order to evaluate a patient's physiologic response to the pulmonary rehabilitation program, it is first necessary to have some common definition of what constitutes an acceptable level of improvement. The term used to describe normal (i.e., nonpulmonary-diseased) individuals is "physical fitness." Physical fitness has been defined as "the ability to maintain certain cardiorespiratory functions as closely as possible to the resting state during strenuous exertion and to restore promptly after exercise any disturbed function."[1] Conventional measurements include changes in heart rate, respiratory rate, minute ventilation, oxygen consumption, CO_2 production, and oxygen cost during exercise and the recovery state. The sum of these would reflect the level of physical fitness so defined.

It would seem plausible to borrow the normal concept of physical fitness and modify it for use in pulmonary rehabilitation language, developing a set of objectives that more succinctly describe the American Thoracic Society's (ATS) baseline definition as cited in the preface of this book. These objectives would then specify within tolerable ranges the physiologic status one should achieve or be capable of achieving once one has completed a pulmonary rehabilitation program. Such a set of objectives would be ideal for the novice as well as the experienced rehabilitation practitioner. It would also give the discipline more specific guidelines to which all could relate. The following objectives suggest guidelines that would allow the practitioner to develop a standard that the patient would be expected to wholly or partially meet. Such objectives are also needed if all the health professionals performing rehabilitative services are to effectively communicate with those agencies (i.e., private pay and commercial insurance and fiscal intermediaries) that dole out the reimbursement for these services. These objectives could act as a working definition of what pulmonary rehabilitation is able to do for the COLD patient.

Not only must one attempt to satisfy third-party payers, but also the legislators who develop the laws governing reimbursement for federally funded medical services. It cannot be overemphasized that a lack of a working definition(s) in the past has led to almost disastrous legislative actions for respiratory care professionals.[2,3] Therefore, the following lists objectives that current pulmonary rehabilitation services should be capable of helping the patient to wholly or partially achieve:

1. Decrease work of breathing and improve ventilation.
2. Improve exercise tolerance.

3. Minimize unnecessary use of accessory muscles or "wasted" breathing efforts by retraining patients in the proper use of diaphragmatic breathing.
4. Teach and emphasize the importance of good bronchopulmonary hygiene.
5. Provide the patient with a basic but thorough understanding of the pathology of the disease process.
6. Provide the patient with information that will help him to recognize and avoid further unnecessary damage to the lungs.
7. Improve self-image and aid in learning to function at optimal physical, emotional, and social levels.
8. Learn physical limitations in regard to the chronicity of disease state.
9. Give emotional, psychosocial, and occupational support and encourage the patient's family to do the same.
10. Stress the importance of performing the various reconditioning exercises at home between outpatient visits.

While it is obvious that COLD patients differ from normal healthy subjects in their response to exercise training, it would be difficult to depict a typical COLD patient who could serve as the physiologic stereotypic model of COLD at any given state of the disease. It would be easier to find a peer group of healthy subjects for comparison with another healthy group than to find even two or three COLD patients with any close compatibility for a similar study. One of the main reasons that it would be difficult to directly compare two COLD patients is that, in addition to the alinear ravages of the disease upon the lungs and body, man ages at different levels and degrees, genetic engineering playing an ever-present role in these processes. Therefore, the clinical or laboratory investigator should keep these factors in mind when attempting to (1) evaluate the clinical state of the disease or (2) measure the effects of pulmonary rehabilitative processes and applying them en masse.

The precise mechanisms by which the beneficial effects of physical training take place are unknown even in the normal subject. The possible mechanisms proposed include better coordination of neuromuscular activity, improved hemodynamic effects, and perhaps increased efficiency of muscular action.[4] The maximal oxygen uptake ($\dot{V}O_2$ max), a reliable guide to improved aerobic capacity in normal subjects, is of limited usefulness in the COLD patient because peak exercise levels are symptom linked at a level below the plateau of the true $\dot{V}O_2$ max. Submaximal exercising may allow the patient to reach a level of exercise that would permit gathering of some useful parameters. A shift in the anaerobic threshold to a higher $\dot{V}O_2$ and decreases in heart rates and ventilatory response at submaximal testing levels may be suggestive of physiologic improvement following extensive pulmonary rehabilitation.[5-8] However, Belman and Wasserman[9] believe that neither of these two methods may yield useful data in the COLD patient with moderate-to-severe obstructive lung disease, because (1) the patient may not be able to even reach anaerobic thresholds, and (2) a decrease in heart rate does not occur in the more severe COLD patient. Thus, we must have other parameters that will more accurately measure the patient's progress. These parameters will be evaluated in two ways: *objective* gains and *subjective* gains.

Evaluating Objective Gains

At first, it would appear to be easy to obtain the objective results of the patient's participation and progress in a pulmonary rehabilitative program: one would merely review the patient's clinical symptoms before and after the program. After all, is this not the process the physician and intensive care unit (ICU) team use in evaluating the patient recovering from an acute (and totally reversible) respiratory crisis requiring ventilator dependence? While it would seem to work with relative mathematical precision in the ICU setting (e.g., blood gas comparison before and after the crisis, tidal volumes before ventilator commitment compared with those present during weaning, etc.), the comparative process does not work that simply when evaluating the long-term COLD patient's progress. The altered pulmonary physiology of the nonchronic lung-diseased patient who has a sudden respiratory crisis is usually short-lived. The expedient attention to the problem by good ICU personnel greatly reduces the likelihood of any serious long-term aftereffects. Conversely, the slow, insidious pathology of COLD is usually not clinically significant in its early stages; therefore, immediate care is sought only after overt clinical symptoms are present, necessitating relief. By this time, the physician will not be able to reverse the disease's pathologic process. Indeed, at this point the physician may only hope to treat the symptoms and prevent the disease from worsening (the antithesis of the ICU scenario above). Equally important is the whole rehabilitation team's ability to recognize which symptoms can be eliminated and which are expected to be tolerable within reasonable ranges. As an example, the very chronicity of the patient's disease creates various long-term physiologic compensatory actions that manifest as a necessary burden (Table 2–1). One of these burdens is the low Pa_{O_2} levels and the usually elevated Pa_{CO_2} levels found in the blood. While these would be poorly tolerated in the nonchronic lung-diseased patient, in the chronically diseased patient these changes are recognized as a new level of homeostasis. Therefore, Pa_{O_2} levels in the low 60s range are tolerable and actually viewed as "normal" for the patient. Likewise, the elevated Pa_{CO_2} levels are "acceptable." In a curious way, these two new levels of blood gas parame-

TABLE 2–1.—COLD PHYSIOLOGIC CHANGES AND
RESULTING FUNCTION*

	ACTION	RESULT
Pa_{O_2}	Decreased	Maintain hypoxic drive
Pa_{CO_2}	Increased	Increased cerebral blood flow
		Oxygen more readily released from blood to tissues due to HbO_2 dissociation curve shifting to right
RBC	Increased	Increased oxygen-carrying capacity of blood

*This table is not meant to imply that these changes are necessarily desirable, but rather that the resulting changes do have an inherent positive value to the COLD patient despite the fact that the change is not "normal" in and of itself.

ters complement each other. The low Pa_{O_2} serves as a constant hypoxic drive mechanism to ensure breathing, while the moderate hypercarbia may assist in improved cerebral circulation. Thus we have a curious symbiosis, but one that may serve the patient well as long as it inadvertently does not shift either way to any great degree.

Healthy individuals are limited not by their lungs, but by their cardiovascular systems. At ambient pressure, the maximal oxygen transport capability of the lungs is more than 6 L of oxygen per minute. The cardiovascular system, conversely, can only carry about 3.8 L of oxygen per minute. Thus, man is normally more limited by his heart and blood capacities than by his lungs. However, this greater pulmonary reserve is brought into balance (or more precisely, imbalance) when COLD takes its toll.

Two common mistakes made when evaluating a COLD patient's response before and after a pulmonary rehabilitation training program are (1) to compare him with a normal, healthy individual and, (2) using and then interpreting physiologic laboratory data that are actually inappropriate for determining progression of the patient's clinical status. A third mistake is the tendency of some physicians and pulmonary rehabilitation evaluators to assess the patient's disability by attempting to quantitate the degree of impairment and expressing it as a percentage of the patient's original or predicted lung function. Such an approach does not take into consideration the natural effects of age, sex, or size and previous state of health to perform a certain work load. For example, a small woman with normal function is not likely to be capable of carrying out certain activities that require great physical strength and effort. Likewise, a 60-year-old man with normal function for his age would probably not be able to carry out many tasks requiring great strength (e.g., heavy lifting) despite the fact that he is otherwise in good cardiopulmonary health.[10]

Table 2–2 compares the objectives of training for both normal individuals and the lung-diseased patient. The contrasts are not only striking, but the beneficial outcome desired for the pulmonary-crippled patient reflect comments made and objectives listed earlier in this chapter regarding fitness for the COLD patient.

Table 2–3 lists the laboratory-measurable physiologic changes that can occur in the patient undergoing pulmonary rehabilitation. These physiologic changes merely represent the more easily measured and clinically significant changes that can possibly occur; they are not meant to be construed as absolute changes, i.e., changes that will definitely occur for all patients and to the same degree. However, when and if these changes do occur, they can be used as part of the documentary evidence required by insurance companies. Table 2–4 lists some criteria for tests. Table 2–5 rates various indices of pulmonary function testing and arterial blood gas analysis.

Evaluating Subjective Gains

New patients entering a pulmonary rehabilitation program are often frightened, anxious, and even depressed due to the physiologic limitations of their disease. Often, as a result of the breathlessness they experience after even minimal physical activity, they self-limit themselves to even a

TABLE 2–2.—OBJECTIVES AND BENEFITS OF A PHYSICAL
TRAINING PROGRAM FOR NORMAL INDIVIDUALS AND
VIGOROUS TREATMENT PROGRAM FOR PULMONARY
PATIENTS*

RESULTS OF PHYSICAL TRAINING IN A NORMAL INDIVIDUAL	RESULTS OF A VIGOROUS TREATMENT PROGRAM FOR A PULMONARY PATIENT
1. Increased maximal oxygen consumption (VO_2 max)	1. Improved exercise tolerance
2. Improved aerobic and anaerobic work capacity	2. Decreased number of severe exacerbations
3. Increased maximal cardiac output and stroke volume	3. Decreased depression and anxiety
4. Decreased resting heart rate	4. Improvement in pulmonary function in patients with reversible components of their airways disease
5. Increased efficiency of distribution of blood during exercise	5. Decrease in premature deaths by reducing episodes of acute respiratory failure
6. Shortening of time required for recovery from exercise	

*From Brashear R.E., Rhodes M.L.: *Chronic Obstructive Lung Disease: Clinical Treatment and Management*, St. Louis, C.V. Mosby Co., 1978, pp. 208–209. Used by permission.

TABLE 2–3.—SUMMARY OF THE EFFECTS OF TRAINING ON CIRCULATORY AND RESPIRATORY FUNCTION DURING PHYSICAL EXERCISE*

VARIABLE	RESPONSE Normal Individual	RESPONSE COLD Individual
Maximal O_2 uptake	Increased	Increased
Work output	Increased	Increased
Mechanical efficiency	Unchanged	Increased slightly
Cardiac output	Increased	Increased
Maximal heart rate	Unchanged	Decreased
Heart rate at submaximal loads	Decreased	Decreased
Stroke volume	Increased	Increased
Arteriovenous O_2 difference	Increased	Increased
Hemoglobin, hematocrit	Unchanged	Decreased slightly or increased with polycythemia
Blood lactate level at maximal loads	Increased	Increased
Blood lactate level at submaximal loads	Decreased	Decreased
Blood flow per unit muscle	Decreased	Decreased
Maximal ventilation	Unchanged	Unchanged
Ventilation at submaximal loads	Decreased	Decreased
Pulmonary diffusing capacity	Unchanged	Unchanged
Capillary density in muscles†	Increased	Increased
Oxidative enzymes in muscles	Increased	Increased

*Adapted from Murray J.: The Normal Lung. Philadelphia, W.B. Saunders Co., 1976.
†Not demonstrated in man.

greater degree of hypostasis. In fact, the patient's reluctance to even slightly tax his physical stamina may add immeasurably to his impairment. This self-imposed hypostasis is as equally the culprit of the patient's misery as are the actual pathologies. The end result physiologically is that the patient's maximum oxygen uptake may be limited by perceived respiratory symptomatologies to a greater degree than what is actually present. Of

TABLE 2–4.—CRITERIA FOR TESTS*

1. Acceptability–safety, discomfort
2. Simplicity–equipment and procedure
3. Objectivity–not influenced by subject cooperation or observer bias
4. Precision (reproducibility) measurement error
   (a) Equipment and observer
   (b) True biological variability
5. Accuracy or validity
   (Relation of quantity measured to what one wishes to know)
   (a) Sensitivity
   (b) Specificity
   (c) Predictive value

*From Morgan W.K.C.: Pulmonary disability and impairment: Can't work? Won't work? Basics of RD 10:5, 1982.[10] Used by permission.

TABLE 2–5.—RATING OF VARIOUS RESPIRATORY FUNCTION TESTS

CRITERIA	FVC‡	FEV$_1$‡	FEF$_{25-75}$‡	PEAK FLOW	V̇MAX$_{50}$‡	V̇MAX$_{75}$‡	LUNG VOLUMES TLC & RV	CV‡	DL$_{CO}$‡	BLOOD GAS DETERMINATIONS	(A – a)O$_2$‡
Acceptability	+++	+++	+++	+++	+++	+++	++	++	++	–	–
Simplicity	+++	+++	+++	++	–	–	–	±	–	–	–
Objectivity	++	++	++	+	++	++	+++	+	+++	+++	–
Reproducibility	+++	+++	– –	++	–	– –	+	±	+++	++	±
Accuracy	++	+++	±	+	±	–	+	–	++	–	±
Sensitivity	+	++	++	+	±	+	– –	++	++	–	+
Specificity	++	+++	–	+	–	–	–	– –	±	– –	–

*Rating system (+ or –) denotes arbitrary positive (+) or negative (–) usefulness of test per criterion.

†From Morgan W.K.C.: Pulmonary disability and impairment: Can't work? Won't work? *Basics of RD* 10:5, 1982.

‡ Definition of abbreviations: FVC = forced vital capacity; FEV$_1$ = forced expiratory volume in one second; FEF$_{25-75}$ = forced expiratory flow during the middle half of the FVC; V̇max$_{50}$ = maximal flow after exhalation of 50% of FVC; V̇max$_{75}$ = maximal flow after exhalation of 75% of FVC; CV = closing volume; DL$_{CO}$ = carbon monoxide diffusing capacity; (A – a)O$_2$ = alveolar-arterial PO$_2$ difference.

course, the various pulmonary testing indices may assist the physician and rehabilitation team in sorting out the real (i.e., objective) from the perceived (i.e., subjective) symptoms.

Nonphysiologic Factors

Chapter 10 will discuss the various psychosocial and other subjective factors that affect the COLD patient's lifestyle. However, as a continuing theme in this book, it would be remiss here to not briefly address some of those factors. The nonphysiologic factors to be considered as an influence on the patient's subjective gains are as follows:

Socioeconomic

The possibility of monetary loss or gain greatly influences a patient's self-assessment of the progress (or regress) made in his pulmonary rehabilitative attempts. For example, the patient with a well-paying job who enjoys his work will be greater motivated to undertake and complete a rehabilitation program. Concomitantly, his compliance may be better. If there are minimal or practically nonexistent socioeconomic resources prior to the patient's illness, then his diagnosis of chronic illness may provide the perfect excuse for an earlier retirement than his disease state would deem necessary. A study by LeRoy-Ladurie and associates[11] found that whereas only 20% of the laboring class return to work after a pneumonectomy, in contrast 70%–89% of the white collar class return. This larger return to work by the professional class is presumed to be partly due to the fact that this group finds greater job interest and monetary incentive to return to work. Another study showed that the total amount of actual respiratory impairment in a group of black lung claimants was less than a group of hospitalized patients who were not claiming any disability.[12] Figure 2–1 plots this relationship.

Psychosocial

The patient's own feelings about himself and where he is at in the self-actualization process will play a significant part in his assessment of benefits to be derived or already gained from a pulmonary rehabilitation program. This is called "self-esteem," and it is not a dynamic process; rather, it is a static one, changing as time goes by and as various situations are encountered. It is further nurtured by the patient's social setting and how he feels he is perceived by significant others in his life. For example, the middle-class, "salt of the earth," hard-working man may be possibly motivated to feel better than what his clinical symptomatology would allow merely because his perceived status is that of the family breadwinner. Such notions can actually be beneficial and greatly augment the therapeutic aspects of

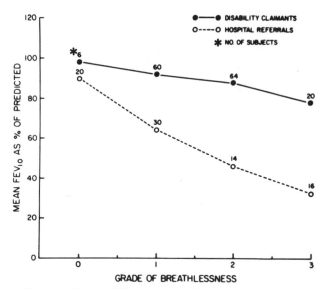

Fig 2–1.—Relationship of FEV$_1$ to grade of breathlessness in a group of 150 coal miners claiming disability, compared with 60 consecutive hospitalized patients. Breathlessness was graded as follows: *0*, none; *1*, more breathlessness than persons of same age while climbing hill or hurrying; *2*, breathless while performing ordinary tasks at work or while walking on level; *3*, shortness of breath at rest or while undressing. (From Morgan W.K.C.: Pulmonary disability and impairment: Can't work? Won't work? *Basics of RD* 10:5, 1982. Used by permission.)

his rehabilitative process, as long as the patient does not allow the perception to be out of proportion to the reality of his clinical status. Chapter 10 will explore psychosocial concepts in depth.

Physiologic Factors

Dyspnea

The best indicator of how the patient feels he is progressing is his self-evaluation of his dyspnea level. While the very nature of dyspnea is one of a perceived degree of breathlessness, there are means by which the patient can be somewhat objectively evaluated at a gross clinical level. The clinician who can ascertain the difference between real (i.e., exercise-induced) or contrived dyspnea has developed an astuteness achieved by few. Table 2–6 quantitates the severity of the patient's dyspnea.

Higher Exercise Tolerance Levels

The patient's unhesitating acceptance to do more and more tasks is one area of improvement that sometimes defies known physiologic standards.

TABLE 2–6.—DEGREE OF SHORTNESS OF
BREATH GRADED FROM 0 TO 4*

GRADE	DESCRIPTION
Grade 0	No shortness of breath with normal activity
	Shortness of breath with exertion, comparable to a well person of the same age, height, and sex.
Grade 1	More shortness of breath than a person of the same age while walking quietly on the level or on climbing an incline or two flights of stairs
Grade 2	More short of breath and unable to keep up with persons of the same age and sex while walking on the level.
Grade 3	Short of breath while walking on the level and while performing everyday tasks at work
Grade 4	Shortness of breath while carrying out personal activities, e.g., dressing, talking, walking from one room to another

*From Morgan, W.K.C.: Pulmonary disability and impairment: Can't work? Won't work? *Basics of RD* 10:5, 1982.[10] Used by permission.

The patient's ability to do more work, as well as a new-found unflagging spirit in which he does it, is most probably due to a modest physiologic improvement and an even greater psychological improvement.

Summary

This chapter has attempted to show the reader the possible objective and subjective gains that a pulmonary rehabilitation program may afford a patient. While both the scientific and empiric observations reported are encouraging, unfortunately there are no hard data replete with exhaustive case studies to document the total effect of pulmonary rehabilitative efforts, nor is there any cookbook approach to assessing the benefits gained by any individual patient. However, these insufficiencies are not to be misconstrued as indicating pulmonary rehabilitation to be an unmeasurable discipline. Instead, pulmonary rehabilitation is a branch of medicine that is in it's infancy stage of art and science, and as such it does not purport to be a discipline of perfect, well-engineered, mathematic precision. As such it would not properly address the human factor with all its inherent frailities, which is the factor for which all of medical science exists.

References

1. Darling R.C.: The significance of physical fitness. *Arch. Phys. Med.* 28:140, 1947.
2. Porte P.: Government policy affecting respiratory therapy, I. *Curr. Rev. Resp. Ther.* 3:44–49, 1980.
3. O'Ryan J.A.: Government policy affecting respiratory therapy, II: Documenting the need for respiratory therapy modalities. *Curr. Rev. Resp. Ther.* 3:50–55, 1980.
4. Pierce A.K., Taylor H.F., Archer R.K.: Responses to exercise training in patients with emphysema. *Arch. Intern. Med.* 113:78–86, 1964.
5. Davis J.A., Frank M.H., Whipp B.J., et al.: Anaerobic threshold alterations caused by endurance training in middle-aged man. *J. Appl. Physiol.: Respiration Environmental Exercise Physiology* 112:219–249, 1979.
6. Astrand P.O., Rodahl K.: *Textbook of Work Physiology: Physiological Bases of Exercise*, ed. 2. New York, McGraw-Hill Book Co., 1977, pp. 391–445.
7. Wasserman K., Whipp B.J., Davis J.A.: Respiratory physiology of exercise: Metabolism, gas exchange and ventilatory control, in Widdicombe J.G. (ed.): *Respiratory Pharmacology*. Section 104: *International Encyclopedia of Pharmacology and Therapeutics*. Oxford, England, Pergamon Press, 1981.
8. Clausen J.P.: Effect of physical training on cardiovascular adjustments to exercise in man. *Physiol. Rev.* 57:779–815, 1977.
9. Belman M.J., Wasserman K.: Exercise training and testing in patients with chronic obstructive pulmonary disease. *Basics of RD* 10:5, 1981.
10. Morgan W.K.C.: Pulmonary disability and impairment: Can't work? Won't work? *Basics Resp. Dis. Am. Lung Assoc.* 10:1–6, 1982.
11. Le Roy-Ladurie M., Silbert D., Ranson-Bitker B.: Facteurs d'invalidité après pneumonectomie. *Bull. Physiopathol. Respir.* 11:182, 1975.
12. Morgan W.K.C.: Disability or disinclination: Impairment or importuning. *Chest* 75:712, 1979.

3 / Pathophysiology of Chronic and Acute Lung Disease

DONALD G. BURNS, D.O.

IN THIS CHAPTER, pathophysiology of the common lung diseases for which rehabilitation is ordered will be discussed. Mention will be made also of methods in rehabilitation by which the pathophysiology may be favorably influenced. Much of the physiology involved in the lung diseases that can be influenced by rehabilitation procedures can only be detected by exercise studies. Patients do not live in a static state, but rather in a dynamic state of exercise. Knowing that the etiology of many pulmonary diseases is environmental and often self-inflicted suggests that these diseases may be prevented or possibly reversed by changes in lifestyle. An attainable goal is a change in lifestyle that may improve the quality of life for these patients.

It should be emphasized that the heart and lungs, although they are separate anatomic entities in the thorax, function as a unitary system for the purpose of gas exchange and tissue perfusion. When either the lungs or heart is stressed, both organs usually respond and are stressed. Abnormalities in either system will impair the delivery of oxygen and the excretion of CO_2. Weakness in the total gas delivery system is the basis for symptoms of cardiopulmonary disease and quite often the target of therapy.[1]

Asthma

Asthma is characterized by episodes of airway obstruction that are usually quite volatile. The hallmark of asthma is the reversibility of the airway obstruction. This reversibility may either occur spontaneously or following treatment. The time necessary for the reversibility of the airway obstruction may vary from a matter of minutes to a matter of weeks. The lungs are relatively normal between attacks. In severe forms of the disease, however, airway resistance may continue to be increased between attacks. The causes of airway obstruction in asthma[2] are (1) inappropriate contraction of the bronchial smooth muscle (bronchospasms), (2) presence of respiratory secretions that are often quite tenacious, and (3) mucosal edema.

17

The exact underlying etiology of asthma is unknown. In the past, much emphasis has been placed on the allergic etiology. Allergy many times does play an important role in asthma; however, it is certainly not the only factor. An immunologic type I reaction between cell-attached IgE or, rarely, IgG and allergin is followed by the release of several chemical substances that bring about the problem of contraction of bronchial smooth muscle as well as mucosal edema. These mediators may also increase respiratory secretions. Mediators released by the mast cells in the lungs, as well as by other routes, are histamine, slow-reacting substance of anaphylaxis (SRSA), serotonin, and prostaglandins. Histamine, prostaglandin F2A, and SRSA are all potent bronchoconstrictors.[3]

Certain precepts regarding the anatomy of the lung should be considered when studying the effect of mediators on airway resistance:

1. Airways down to the terminal bronchioles are innervated by the vagus nerve and perfused by the bronchial arteries.
2. The airways beyond the terminal bronchioles, which include the alveolar ducts and respiratory bronchioles, contain smooth muscle; however, they are not innervated by the vagus and are perfused by the pulmonary circulation rather than the bronchial circulation.[4]
3. Many of the bronchoactive substances including prostaglandins El, E2, and F2A as well as serotonin, acetylcholine, and bradykinin are almost entirely removed from the venous blood by the lung in a single passage. Histamine is not removed by the lung in this way.[5]

From the above precepts, it can be seen that different substances may have varying effects, depending on whether they are inhaled or delivered in the mixed venous or bronchial blood. The following categories summarize the more significant physiologic activities ocurring in asthma:

Histamine

Histamine is released after a type I IgE reaction. Antihistamines have been found to be of little use in the treatment of asthma.

Histamine injected into the bronchial arteries of dogs causes construction of the innervated trachea down to the area of the terminal bronchioles. This causes a large rise in the airway resistance and minimal change in compliance of the lung. This effect of histamine can be blocked by vagotomy.

Injection of histamine into the pulmonary arteries of dogs also caused an immediate constriction of the respiratory bronchioles and alveolar ducts, with a minimal rise in resistance. This is due to the fact that these airways make up a small fraction of the total resistance of the lung. A large fall in compliance was noted. This effect was not altered by vagotomy. Injecting antihistamines prior to the injection of histamine into the dogs' pulmonary arteries or bronchial arteries would block the effect on the lung.[4] This does not occur in clinical asthma. It is unknown whether this is due to the fact that histamine is not important in the pathogenesis of asthma or possibly because locally released histamine cannot be blocked.

Histamine not only causes contraction of the smooth muscles in the bronchial wall, but also considerable edema. This appears to be secondary to an increased permeability in the vessels. This is largely restricted to the bronchial venules.

Serotonin

Serotonin causes peripheral bronchial and alveolar duct constriction as well as large airway constriction. Serotonin does not seem to affect bronchial venular permeability.[6]

Bradykinin

Bradykinin, when infused intravenously (IV) in man, does not cause significant change in resistance in either large or small airways. It does cause a fall in vital capacity, suggesting that there may be alveolar duct constriction.[7]

SRSA

The relevance of this substance in clinical asthma is unknown at this time.

Prostaglandins

Asthmatic patients are very sensitive to prostaglandins and may have severe bronchoconstriction with minute doses of prostaglandin F2A. They may react to approximately $\frac{1}{10,000}$ of the dose that gives a measurable reaction in normal individuals.[8] A type I IgE reaction causes release of both prostaglandin F2A as well as prostaglandins E1 and E2. Both E1 and E2 are bronchodilators; at the present time, the relative proportions of the two released are unknown. This may vary from patient to patient and may account for the fact that while some patients' asthma is apparently improved by aspirin, others may have a severe exacerbation of asthma with aspirin.

Cyclic Adenosine Monophosphate

Asthmatic patients following an injection of epinephrine have a lesser output of cyclic adenosine monophosphate (CAMP) in the urine than normal individuals.[9] It has also been noted that leukocytes and lymphocytes from patients with asthma have a decreased concentration of CAMP.[10]

The patients with asthma often behave as if they were in a continuous partial state of beta adrenergic blockade. Evidence of autonomic dysfunction in asthmatics is suggested. There is data to point to excess cholinergic responsiveness such as altered sweat responses and the reversal of antigen-induced bronchospasm by atropine.[11]

Other neural contributions to asthma may be present. The "irritant" receptors of the lungs are indicated in asthmatic patients by the onset of hyperventilation soon after antigen exposure but before the patient has apparent bronchospasm.

Exercise-induced asthma is poorly understood from the pathophysiologic standpoint. It has been found that the stimuli that lead to airway cooling cause bronchospasm in susceptible individuals. The basic problem appears to be the heat transfer. Hyperventilation or breathing cold, dry air may cause an exacerbation of asthma.

Alterations in Mechanics and Gas Exchange

Regardless of the underlying etiology of asthma, the abnormalities that occur in the lung function are similar. The airway resistance is increased in asthma and leads to increased airway pressure. The resistance increase is thought to be due to a multitude of factors including bronchoconstriction as well as mucosal edema and inspissated secretions.

The residual volume and total lung capacity in asthma is increased. This increase occurs rapidly following an inhalation challenge of antigen. Reduced flow rates and probably decreased elastic recoil, as well as early airway closure, may ensue. Decreased muscle power may also be a factor in the increase in total lung capacity early in an asthma attack.

An acute asthma attack is generally accompanied by abnormalities in gas exchange including hypoxemia as well as hypocarbia with its resultant respiratory alkalosis. The hypoxemia seems to be related to the airflow obstruction. This is apparently due to ventilation perfusion inequality. Gas exchange may also be affected by the pattern of ventilation. Hyperventilation, perhaps mediated by neurologic factors, often accompanies an acute asthma attack. Following treatment of the attack, the patient's hypoxemia is often slow to respond, not improving until long after lung mechanics improvement is seen. This is apparently due to persistent small airway obstruction and resulting ventilation perfusion inequality.

During an asthma attack, hypoxic vasoconstriction and redistribution of pulmonary blood flow often take place. Some bronchodilators may actually increase the blood flow and reduce the hypoxic vasoconstriction, causing increased ventilation perfusion inequalities and exacerbation of hypoxemia. See Table 3–1 for a summary of the physiologic factors in asthma.

TABLE 3–1.—SUMMARY OF PHYSIOLOGIC FACTORS IN
ASTHMA

MECHANICS
   1. Total lung capacity increased
   2. Residual volume increased
   3. Decreased muscle power
   4. Decreased flow rates
GAS EXCHANGE
   1. Hypoxemia due to abnormal ventilation/perfusion relationships
   2. Hypocarbia due to neurologic mediated hyperventilation

Emphysema

The Greek origin of the word emphysema is a term meaning inflation.[3] Although lung tissue involved by emphysema is frequently overinflated, the essential criterion for the diagnosis of pulmonary emphysema is the destruction of the interalveolar septa. Emphysema is defined in anatomic terms as an abnormal and permanent enlargement of the airspaces distal to the terminal bronchioles accompanied by destruction of their wall. Emphysema is, therefore, a disease of the terminal respiratory units. Pure emphysema rarely exists alone; virtually all patients have associated chronic bronchitis and, at times bronchiectasis and asthma. The following four areas summarize the anatomic changes that occur in emphysema:

Lung Volumes

The changes in lung volumes in pure emphysema are secondary to the loss of elastic recoil of the diseased lungs. Mechanical properties of the respiratory system differ from those of normal subjects. The total lung capacity is increased secondary to the usual inspiratory muscle forces, causing the weakened lungs to contain a larger than normal volume of air. The functional residual capacity is increased because of the loss of inward recoil of the lungs, offering less opposition to the outward recoil of the chest wall. Residual volume is increased because of loss of recoil and tethering of the airways. This causes them to close prematurely. Generally, the vital capacity is nearly normal, because the increase in residual volume is partially offset by the increase in total lung capacity.

Mechanics of Ventilation

Decreased airflow is present in pulmonary emphysema secondary to decreased elastic recoil. The airflow is decreased at all lung volumes because the elastic recoil is decreased at all lung volumes. In patients with emphysema, the equal pressure point at which pleural pressure equals endobronchial pressure moves peripherally from the central large bronchi to the more peripheral airways. This exposes the tracheobronchial system to dynamic compression.

Gas Exchange

The alveolar-capillary surface for gas exchange is decreased in pulmonary emphysema due to destruction of the interalveolar septa. This is reflected by a decreased diffusing capacity of the lung for both oxygen and CO_2. Not all pulmonary capillaries are perfused in normal persons under resting conditions; therefore, extra pathways are ordinarily present that can accommodate increased blood flow during exercise. These extra pathways are available in case some channels are destroyed or obstructed. It can, therefore, be suggested that a small amount of emphysema can occur without affecting measurements of diffusing capacity at rest, because blood flow simply shifts from the obliterated to the other available capillaries. During exercise, the diffusing capacity does not increase as much as in a normal individual, because these spare pathways are already being utilized.

In patients with severe emphysema, many times the P_{O_2} is only slightly decreased. This is because most of the cardiac output is distributed to units with slightly lower-than-normal ventilation perfusion ratios. There is very little blood flow to units of very low ventilation perfusion ratios or to right-to-left shunts. In contrast to the pattern of distribution of blood flow, a large fraction of ventilation is distributed to regions with high ventilation perfusion ratios. This is caused by destruction of lung parenchyma in emphysema. The decrease in elastic recoil makes the involved units more easily ventilated, whereas the loss of capillaries decreases their perfusion. Arterial CO_2 values are usually normal in patients with emphysema, even in advanced stages. This finding may seem surprising in the presence of severe obstruction to airflow. This is readily explained by the fact that there is some CO_2 elimination from the regions that are well ventilated but poorly perfused. This effect offsets the mild tendency for arterial CO_2 to increase from the extensive perfusion of regions with slightly lower-than-normal ventilation perfusion ratios. These patients, however, must increase the minute volume of ventilation to make up for the large fraction of inspired air that contributes little or nothing to gas exchange.

Predictions of arterial P_{O_2} values from observed distributions of ventilation and blood flow agree with direct measurements. The agreement between the predicted and measured values reinforces the fact that despite severe decreases in diffusing capacity, limitations of diffusion are not an important cause of arterial hypoxia in these patients. In pulmonary emphysema, the distribution during exercise of ventilation and perfusion is essentially the same as that at rest. Because of this, the low P_{O_2} cannot be fully explained by worsened ventilation/perfusion mismatching or diffusing abnormalities. This implies that oxygen consumption during exercise increases proportionally more than cardiac output and that the venous-arterial difference widens, thereby causing a drop in the arterial oxygen level.

Control of Breathing

The important differences between eucapnic and hypercapnic patients with obstructive pulmonary disease are that the former have greater increased diaphragmatic electrical activity during CO_2 breathing than the latter.[12] Increased drive to breathe and increased muscle activity undoubtedly help the emphysema patient maintain the normal arterial oxygen level until quite late in his disease. Table 3–2 summarizes the physiologic factors in emphysema.

Chronic Bronchitis

Chronic bronchitis is defined in clinical terms. However, the pathology is now well documented. The bronchitic patient has excessive production of mucus, usually with recurrent cough and expectoration. The clinical definition is that the patient must be symptomatic on most days for at least 3 months per year during a period of 2 successive years. Other causes of increased sputum production must be eliminated, such as bronchiectasis or tuberculosis.[3] The pathologic changes due to chronic bronchitis are summarized here.

Lung Volumes

The total lung capacity in the purely bronchitic patient is generally normal. The elastic recoil of the lungs and chest wall also appears to be essentially normal. The major abnormality in chronic bronchitis is that of an

TABLE 3–2.— SUMMARY OF PHYSIOLOGIC FACTORS IN EMPHYSEMA

LUNG VOLUMES
1. Total lung capacity increased
2. Residual volume increased
3. Functional residual volume increased
4. Vital capacity normal
5. Elastic recoil decreased

MECHANICS
1. Dystonia of airways
2. Decreased airflow at all lung volumes
3. Equal pressure point moves peripheral in airways with early airway closure

GAS EXCHANGE
1. Alveolar capillary surface decreased
2. Eucapnia until late
3. Normal P_{O_2} early in emphysema

CONTROL OF BREATHING
Hyperpnea with CO_2 breathing

increased residual volume that reflects premature closure of the narrowed airways during expiration. This situation is analogous in part to that of patients with asthma, where the airways also close prematurely.

Mechanics of Ventilation

In the chronic bronchitic with normal elastic recoil, decreased maximal expiratory flow is caused by increased resistance of the upstream airway. This agrees with the pathologic findings in chronic bronchitis.

Gas Exchange

These patients generally have a relatively normal diffusing capacity. This correlates with the fact that in chronic bronchitis, the alveolar capillary surface for gas exchange is intact. The chronic bronchitic patient characteristically has low values for arterial oxygen, and this is secondary to abnormal ventilation perfusion ratios. In these patients a large fraction of the cardiac output is distributed to regions where the ventilation perfusion ratios are markedly decreased. The hypercapnia present in the chronic bronchitic patient causes no particular change in the distribution of ventilation perfusion. Generally, severe alveolar hypoxia causes a decrease in blood flow to these areas. This finding would suggest that the hypoxic vasoconstrictor mechanism is inoperative or overwhelmed in these particular patients.

Control of Breathing

The ventilatory response to hypercapnia is decreased in nearly all patients with chronic bronchitis. Hypercapnic patients have a decreased drive to breathe, and the arterial CO_2 values correlate better with ventilatory drive than with the abnormal mechanics. The reasons for this decreased respiratory drive are not known. The increased buffering capacity from increases in bicarbonate in blood and cerebral spinal fluid mask some of the effect of increases in arterial CO_2 on pH. This is not a completely satisfactory explanation. A more likely theory holds that the patients are poor responders to chemical stimuli because of genetic predisposition. It is also possible that some loss of drive can be acquired by mechanisms similar to those that account for acquired loss of chemoreceptor resensitivity that has been documented in long-term residence at high altitude.[12] Table 3–3 summarizes the factors operative in chronic bronchitis.

Fatigue of the Diaphragm

The inspiratory muscles of the respiration can generally sustain breathing for life without fatigue. The normal diaphragm will fatigue only when the work of breathing is severely increased by external ventilatory loads. Dur-

TABLE 3–3.—SUMMARY OF PHYSIOLOGIC FACTORS
IN CHRONIC BRONCHITIS

LUNG VOLUMES
  1. Total lung capacity normal
  2. Elastic recoil normal
  3. Residual volume increased
  4. Vital capacity decreased
MECHANICS
  Increased resistance in large bronchi
GAS EXCHANGE
  1. Diffusing capacity near normal
  2. Decreased ventilation/perfusion ratios and hypoxemia
CONTROL OF BREATHING
  Decreased drive to breathe with CO_2 breathing

ing neuromuscular disease, the diaphragm may be weakened either by denervation or by pathologic processes that involve the diaphragm itself. The diaphragm is rendered more susceptible to fatigue in a variety of ways. This includes the decreased work of breathing as well as decreased mechanical advantage, alterations in neurologic drive, and metabolic structural changes that adversely affect the contractility of the inspiratory muscles. Fatigue of the diaphragm and other inspiratory muscles is clinically important, because it leads to dyspnea, compromises exercise performance, and contributes to the development of respiratory failure.

Two types of fatigue have been categorized, according to origin, as *central* and *peripheral*. Central fatigue is a consequence of inadequate neurodrive, as in nervous system disease. Peripheral fatigue is secondary to abnormalities in the muscle itself. While fatigue of both expiratory and inspiratory muscles undoubtedly occurs, the dominant role of the inspiratory muscles in sustaining breathing has led investigators to focus on this group.[13]

The adult human diaphragm is made up of approximately 55% of the fibers of the slow twitch type, which have a high oxidative and low glycolytic capacity. These muscle fibers are highly resistant to fatigue. Approximately 20% are fast twitch type red fibers that have high oxidative and glycolytic capacity. These fibers are also quite resistant to fatigue. The remaining 25% are fast twitch white fibers with high glycolytic but low oxidative capacity.[14] These 25% of the fibers are those most susceptible to fatigue (Table 3–4). The high percentage of fibers with high endurance properties have approximately three times as many capillaries and four times the volume of mitochondria per unit volume of muscle as limb skeletal muscle.[15] Animal studies have shown that during high levels of contractile force and energy expenditure, the diaphragmatic blood flow may increase up to 25 times the level of perfusion during quiet breathing. The

TABLE 3–4.—PROPERTIES OF MUSCLE FIBER TYPES

	FIBER		
	I	IIA	IIB
Color	Intermediate	Red	White
Twitch type	Slow	Fast	Fast
Endurance	Excellent	Good	Poor
Oxidative capacity	High	High	Low
Glycolytic capacity	Low	Intermediate	High
% in diaphragm	55%	20%	25%

oxygen requirements for the diaphragm are met primarily by increasing blood flow, whereas limb skeletal muscle, blood flow, and oxygen extraction initially increase together. In work rates in excess of 60% of the maximum blood flow, the action requirements can only be met by further increasing oxygen extraction. In the presence of inspiratory resistance, the increase in diaphragmatic blood flow is about 25-fold, which is three times as much as in the external intercostal muscles and about 10 times as much as in the scalene muscles.[15] It can be seen from these studies that the diaphragm appears to supply a majority of the power to overcome resistance and maintain ventilation.

Because of the increase in airway resistance in hyperinflation of the lungs, the increase in work and energy cost of breathing often goes to extraordinary levels. The inspiratory work in the presence of obstructive pulmonary disease is elevated by two mechanisms: (1) increased resistance to inspiratory flow and (2) increased elastic work to stretch the lung at high-lung volumes and the timing of inspiratory muscle contraction.

There is circumstantial evidence that acute fatigue of the normal diaphragm is injurious. The diaphragm does not recover from low-frequency fatigue for 12 to 24 hours.[16] Animal studies have demonstrated that severe injury to the skeletal muscle fibers is associated with activation of the lysosomal system. This becomes evident pathologically usually within 5 days after an exhaustive run.[17] However, in animals that have been preconditioned by exercise training, only minimal muscle damage occurs after fatigue of the skeletal muscles. Similar observations do not exist with the diaphragm, although it has been noted that serum levels of muscle creatine kinase are elevated during an acute attack of asthma.[17]

Disuse atrophy damages contractile elements of limb skeletal muscle. The nutritional status also appears to be important in that a decrease in body weight to 70% of ideal is accompanied by approximately a 40% reduction in diaphragm muscle mass.[18] Chronic disease also renders transmembrane potentials of skeletal muscles about 25% less negative than normal, and the sodium intracellular concentration is increased by 42%.[19]

These changes may suggest compromises of the sarcolemmal membrane and/or the sodium potassium adenosine triphosphatase pump mechanism. It is noted that hypophosphatemia may also lead to severe muscle weakness and acute respiratory failure. Hypophosphatemia also affects muscle membrane function.

Although the airflow resistance is more increased during expiration than inspiration, the increase in ventilatory work is affected primarily by the inspiratory muscles which, because of the increased lung volumes, are operating at a mechanical disadvantage.

Pulmonary Rehabilitation Considerations

Rehabilitation of the patient with acute and chronic lung diseases should involve as much as possible a reversal of the factors that are contributing to the etiology of the disease. It appears at this time that a common etiologic factor in the development of chronic bronchitis and emphysema is cigarette smoking; therefore the rehabilitation program should be directed toward elimination of this self-destructive habit. Exposure to dust and irritating factors to the bronchi should also be minimized as much as possible.

The exact etiology in asthma is unknown; however, many patients have exacerbations due to known factors such as allergy. Exposure to these factors should also be minimized and the patient educated as to methods of avoidance of specific exacerbating factors.

Panic Training

Panic training is a technique that involves training the patient in relaxation during dyspneic episodes. At times, the asthmatic may be able to abort an attack by simple relaxation techniques. Relaxation also allows the patient to breathe at lower flow rates, thereby decreasing turbulence in the airways, and allowing more laminar airflow with better peripheral ventilation. The training techniques usually involve some biofeedback-type mechanism that will allow the patient to realize when relaxation is not occurring.

Education of the patient regarding disease processes will also enable him to relax during an acute episode of symptomatology and allow a decreased oxygen consumption. Understanding the mechanisms of his disease will help to remove the patient's fear of the unknown. Chapter 6 discusses biofeedback in depth.

Decrease of Work of Breathing

Teaching the patient to breath in a more mechanically efficient method may decrease the work of breathing, thereby decreasing oxygen consumption and the CO_2 load that must be eliminated by the lungs. Improving bronchial hygiene, and thus decreasing the amount of secretions in the lungs, may also decrease the resistive load that increases the work of breathing. Improving the patient's nutritional status may improve inspiratory muscle function. By manipulating the diet, the CO_2 production may also be affected, which is helpful in reducing the demands on the ventilatory capacity for removal of CO_2.

Inspiratory Muscle Fatigue

One of the most common causes for hospitalization in the COLD patient is acute respiratory failure secondary to inspiratory muscle fatigue. Once the fatigue has occurred, there are several techniques that may be helpful in reducing it.

The first approach to treating muscle fatigue is rest. The rationale for rest therapy is to allow the muscle membrane time to recover from the abnormalities that characterize both high- and low-frequency fatigue. Rest also permits the inspiratory muscles to recover depleted energy stores. Contributing factors such as water and electrolyte imbalance, infection, fever, hypophosphatemia, and nutritional impairment should be corrected so the inspiratory muscles are in optimal shape to resume their ventilatory task. If the fatigue has already set in, it is usually necessary to place the patient on mechanical ventilation and maintain ventilator assistance for at least 12 to 24 hours until the inspiratory muscles have a chance to recover. In patients who are especially susceptible to inspiratory muscle fatigue, prophylactic techniques such as the use of body respirators for a period of 8 to 16 hours daily may be helpful.[20] For these short periods of time, it is unlikely that disuse atrophy of the inspiratory muscles will occur because the patient is exercising the inspiratory muscles for several hours each day.

A second approach to the treatment of inspiratory muscle fatigue is the use of drugs. It has been demonstrated that a contractile force for any given level of electrical stimulation is increased by use of aminophylline. Pretreatment with aminophylline shortens the duration of fatigue, and administration of aminophylline after fatigue develops restores the force to normal after approximately 20 minutes.[21] Aminophylline appears to rapidly reverse low-frequency fatigue, which is particularly detrimental to inspiratory muscle performance.[21] How long the aminophylline effect lasts or whether it can reverse fatigue in the inspiratory muscles of chronically ill patients has not been established.[21]

A third approach to treating inspiratory muscle fatigue is muscle training. This not only increases the proportion of fatigue-resistant fibers in the diaphragm, but reduces the susceptibility of these fibers to the destructive effects of exhaustive exercise.[13] Endurance training improves inspiratory muscle performance, as demonstrated by increases in critical level of inspiratory pressure, as well as improving maximum sustained ventilation and forestalling the onset of fatigue.

Enhancement of inspiratory muscle endurance may be carried out by an inspiratory training regime and must involve repeated rhythmic inspiratory efforts. Some of these regimes involve maximum voluntary ventilation maneuvers. A useful regime is that based on inspiratory resistive loading. Commercial devices are now available through which the patient may carry out these exercises several times a day (see Chapter 5). In order to be effective, this inspiratory endurance training must be practiced several times a day for at least 4 to 5 days per week. The enhanced ventilatory performance is usually demonstrated by 6 weeks of training; however, further improvement occurs when the regime is prolonged to 12 weeks.[17] It is still uncertain what an optimum regime is and how much work is needed to maintain the benefits after the initial training period.

Aerobic-type training is also helpful in that it may reduce the oxygen comsumption for a given level of work. This may allow the patient to be more active during his daily activities. Aerobic-type walking or swimming exercises may also improve inspiratory muscle function, apparently by the maximum voluntary ventilation obtained during these exercises.

Summary

The basic pathophysiology of COLD involves that of increased resistance to airflow. Secondary to this is hyperinflation of the lung with resultant mechanical disadvantage to the inspiratory muscles. This ultimately causes shortening of the muscle fibers of the diaphragm, allowing for early development of inspiratory muscle fatigue. Many of the patients with chronic obstructive pulmonary disease are also in a state of poor nutrition, which further predisposes one to fatigue of the inspiratory muscles.

Abnormalities in the control of ventilation also occur in COLD and predispose the patient to the ravages of respiratory acidosis. The primary disease process in the lung, as well as the vasoconstrictive influences of acidosis, hypoxemia, and hypercapnia, cause pulmonary hypertension and its resultant effect on the right ventricle.

Rehabilitative techniques in COLD treatment involve techniques for decreasing work of respiration through improving mechanical abnormalities as well as decreasing oxygen consumption and CO_2 production for a given amount of work. Treatment of inspiratory muscle fatigue involves resting the inspiratory muscles as well as utilization of aminophylline to reverse acute diaphragmatic fatigue. Metabolic abnormalities must be corrected by administering oxygen and correcting electrolyte imbalance and hypophosphatemia. Improvement in the nutritional status is necessary in the treatment and prophylaxis of inspiratory muscle fatigue. Inspiratory muscle endurance training also increases the proportion of fatigue-resistant fibers of the diaphragm, offering considerable promise for long-term management.

References

1. Wilson P.K.: *Rehabilitation of the Heart and Lungs,* ed. 1. Fullerton, Calif.: Beckman Instruments Inc., 1980.
2. Kiss G.T.: *Diagnosis and Management of Pulmonary Disease,* ed. 1. Menlo Park, Calif.: Addison-Wesley Publishing Co., 1982.
3. Smith L.H.: *Pathophysiology,* ed. 1. Philadelphia: W.B. Saunders Co., 1981.
4. Saunders K.B.: *Clinical Physiology of the Lung,* ed. 1. Oxford, England, Blackwell Scientific Publications, 1977.
5. Vane J.R.: The release and fate of vaso-active hormones in the circulation. *Br. Med. J.* 1:15, 1969.
6. Colebatch H.J.H., Olsen C.R., Nadel J.A.: Effect of histamine, serotonin and acetylcholine on the peripheral airways. *J. Appl. Physiol.* 21:217, 1966.
7. Newball H.H., Kaiser H.R.: Relative effects of bradykinin and histamine on the respiratory system of man. *J. Appl. Physiol.* 35:552–556, 1973.
8. Mathe A.R., Hedquist P., Holmgren A., et al.: Bronchial hyperreactivity to prostaglandin F_{2a} and histamine with asthma. *Br. Med. J.* 1:193, 1973.
9. Bernstein R.A., Linarelli L., Facktor M.A., et al.: Decreased urinary adenosine 3', 5' monophosphate (cyclic AMO) in asthmatics. *J. Lab. Clin. Med.* 80:722, 1972.
10. Parker C.W., Smith J.W.: Alterations in cyclic adenosine monophosphate metabolism in human bronchial asthma: Leucocyte responsiveness to B-adrenergic agents. *J. Clin. Invest.* 52:48, 1973.
11. Yu D.Y.C., Galant S.P., Gold W.M.: Inhibition of antigen induced bronchoconstriction by atropine in asthmatic patients. *J. Appl. Physiol.* 32:823, 1972.
12. Altose M.D., McCauley W.C., Kelson S.G., et al.: Effects of hypercapnia and inspiratory flow resistive loading on respiratory activity in chronic airway obstruction. *J. Clin. Invest.* 59:500, 1977.
13. Edwards R.H.T.: The diaphragm as a muscle: Contractile properties. *Am. Rev. Respir. Dis.* 119 (suppl.):89, 1979.
14. Faulkner J.A., Maxwell L.C., Ruff G.L., et al.: The diaphragm as a muscle: Contractile properties. *Am. Rev. Respir. Dis.* 119 (suppl.):89, 1979.
15. Robertson C.H., Foster G.H., Johnson R.L. Jr.: The relationship of respiratory failure to the oxygen consumption of, lactate production by, and distribution of blood flow among respiratory muscles during increasing inspiratory resistance. *J. Clin. Invest.* 59:31, 1977.
16. Edwards R.H.T.: The diaphragm as a muscle: Mechanisms underlying fatigue. *Am. Rev. Respir. Dis.* 119(suppl.): 81, 1979.
17. Fishman A.P.: *Update: Pulmonary Diseases and Disorders,* ed. 1. New York, McGraw-Hill Book Co., 1982.
18. Thurlbeck W.M.: Diaphragm and body weight on emphysema. *Thorax* 33:483, 1978.
19. Cunningham J.N. Jr., Carter N.W., Rector F.C. Jr., et al.: Resting transmembrane potential difference of skeletal muscle in normal subjects and severely ill patients. *J. Clin. Invest.* 50:49, 1971.

20. Rochester D.F., Braun N.M.T., Laine S.: Diaphragmatic energy expenditure in chronic respiratory failure: The effect of assisted ventilation with body respirators. *Am. J. Med.* 63:223, 1977.
21. Aubier M., DeTroyer A., Sampson M., et al.: Aminophylline improves diaphragmatic contractility in man. *N. Engl. J. Med.* 305:249, 1981.

4 / Diagnostic Techniques for Assessing Pulmonary Dysfunction

DONALD G. BURNS, D.O.

PULMONARY DYSFUNCTION may be classified into several types based on patterns of abnormalities and physiologic response. Abnormalities in response can be detected by numerous techniques. One of the most useful techniques is that of obtaining an in-depth and accurate history of the patient's symptoms. An equally useful technique is that of performing a physical examination. Many of the abnormalities that occur in physiology can be detected by observation of the patient as well as by auscultation of the patient's lungs. Palpation and percussion are also essential parts of the physical examination. Certain laboratory data may be helpful in evaluation of the patient's physiology. The blood count, as well as examination of the sputum, may be extremely helpful. Blood chemistry analysis is also useful in ascertaining either the etiology of the patient's problem or the effects of the disease on the patient's physiology. The electrocardiogram (ECG) is of obvious importance in evaluation of the patient's physiology. This is helpful in determining cor pulmonale late in the patient with chronic obstructive lung disease (COLD). Chest radiographs are also important in ascertaining anatomic changes that have occurred in the patient's chest. Pulmonary function studies, including spirographic testing as well as lung volume determinations and diffusing capacity, should be performed. One of the most useful tests is that of exercise testing in determining the patient's physiologic response to activity.

History

The symptoms that an individual experiences depend on various factors. The abnormalities in function themselves may produce symptomatology. Compensatory mechanisms to the abnormality in function may also cause certain symptoms.

People vary in their perception of abnormalities. A common occurrence during history taking is denial of certain symptoms by the patient. Even during the denial, the physician may note that the patient is experiencing the symptom. An example of this is cough or wheezing. This has led us to develop and depend on more objective data.

The main pulmonary symptoms that the examiner must obtain during the history-taking process are those of dyspnea, cough, hemoptysis, wheezing, and chest pain.[1] In questioning the patient regarding these symptoms, it is important to determine the length of time the symptoms have been present as well as their severity. It is also important to elicit any aggravating factors as well as factors that seem to relieve the symptoms. At times, it is useful to determine if the patient's symptomatology is out of proportion to their obvious physical condition. It is also important to note if the patient's exercise tolerance is different from that of his peers when undertaking the same level of activity.

Often the symptomatology secondary to lung disease is essentially that found in cardiac disease. Confirmatory evidence of heart disease, however, can almost always be found by physical examination, chest x-ray examination, or ECG examination.

Other important factors to determine during the history-taking process are occupational or environmental exposures that the patient may have had. It is important to determine when the exposure occurred. Problems such as asbestosis may have a lag period between the initial exposure and the development of pulmonary disease. An example of this is development of bronchogenic carcinoma following asbestos exposure. This may have a latent period of up to 20 years.

The patient's family history may also be important not only in determining certain hereditary diseases, but also in determining certain infectious diseases. A history of tuberculosis in family or close associates should be determined.

Obtaining an in-depth history regarding symptoms in other systems is essential. Many times, disease processes that involve other systems may also have an effect on the lungs. Examples of this may include immunologic diseases, diseases of the upper respiratory tract, and gastrointestinal diseases. Reversible obstructive airway disease may be secondary to aspiration of stomach contents secondary to gastroesophageal incompetence.

The smoking history should also be examined in detail. The amount of tobacco smoked is important as well as the duration of smoking. This may be expressed as "pack-years." It may also be useful to determine the pattern of smoking. An example of this is whether the patient usually smokes only half of the cigarette or whether it is smoked down to a very short butt. The patient's inhalation pattern should also be noted.

The past history should be ascertained. It is important to know if the patient has had recurrent episodes of pulmonary infections. It is useful to know the childhood history of the patient, because some of the diseases such as measles or adenoviral infections may later cause severe problems such as bronchiectasis.

Physical Examination

One of the most useful methods of examination of the patient is observation. The pattern of respiration and frequency may be observed with the patient at rest as well as on exercise. The patient's use of accessory muscles of respirations should be observed. The shape of the chest gives helpful information. Malformations of the bony thorax and spine, such as pectus excavatum, pigeon chest, kyphosis, scoliosis, and lordosis, should be noted.

Palpation of the neck is helpful in determining if tracheal deviation is present. Palpation of the fingers may suggest sponginess at the fixed end of the nail plate. This is an early sign of clubbing and may be associated with hypertrophic pulmonary osteoarthropathy. Palpation of the abdomen is also useful in that a low-lying liver is common with an individual with hyperinflation of the lungs. One may also be able to palpate the left parasternal lift with a right ventricular hypertrophy often occurring in late cor pulmonale.

A common physical finding in airway obstruction that seems to correlate best with pulmonary function is the time of forced expiration. The individual is asked to fill his lungs as completely as possible and then with an open mouth expire their air as rapidly as possible. Normal emptying time of the lungs is approximately 3 to 4 seconds. If the emptying time is greater than 6 to 7 seconds, the patient probably has significant obstruction of the airways.

Auscultation of the chest is useful in helping to determine physiologic abnormalities. Wheezing is a common symptom noted when the patient's airflow is around 30% of predicted. This wheezing generally disappears when the patient improves to 50% of predicted airflow or better. The wheezing may also disappear if airflows fall to extremely low levels.[2]

The remainder of the physical examination may provide clues to the etiology of the dyspnea, cough, or other symptomatology in the pulmonary patient. Collateral vessels can be seen across the chest in superior vena caval obstruction. It is possible to palpate nodules in the liver in the patient with metastatic bronchogenic carcinoma. Numerous neurologic findings including mononeuropathy, polyneuropathy, and corticocerebellar degeneration may be noted in patients with abnormal blood gases or with bronchogenic metastasis.

Laboratory Data

The complete blood count may be useful in determining problems in the pulmonary patient.[3] The patient's hemoglobin may be reduced, which thereby reduces the oxygen-carrying capacity. This can be a primary cause of dyspnea. The finding of erythrocytosis may suggest that the patient has hypoxemia, either intermittent or continuous. The white blood cell count can be suggestive of the presence of bacterial or viral infections. A high eosinophil count may indicate asthma or, at times, hypersensitivity disease.

Observation, as well as culture and cytologic examination of the sputum, is helpful in ascertaining the etiology of the patient's pulmonary problem. Microscopic examination of the sputum either in the unstained or stained preparation will help to identify cell types as well as bacteria in sputum. The gross appearance of the sputum also is helpful. The presence of neutrophils, as well as eosinophils, gives the sputum a purulent appearance.

Blood chemistry analysis may be a diagnostic aid in evaluating the patient with pulmonary disease. Protein electrophoresis may reveal α_1-antitrypsin deficiency. Immunoglobulin levels are suggested in the patient with recurrent infection.

Chest X-ray

Diagnostic x-rays of the chest are important in evaluation of the patient with respiratory complaints. Anatomic changes with infiltrates, masses, or changes in the pulmonary volume may be observed. Mediastinal disease causing pulmonary symptoms also can be determined.

The effectiveness of the chest x-ray in establishing a diagnosis of emphysema is somewhat limited, because this diagnosis can rarely be made on the radiologic appearance alone.[4] The classic radiologic changes of emphysema are increased radiolucency with bullae and decreased peripheral pulmonary vasculature. The retrosternal airspace on the lateral film may be increased. The diaphragms are often low and flattened. Inspiratory and expiratory films often reveal a movement of less than 3 cm of the diaphragm. Normally the diaphragm should move at least 5 cm on a maximum inspiration and expiration. Often the heart is vertical and appears small. The pulmonary arteries and right ventricle may be quite prominent. If these findings are present, advanced pulmonary obstructive disease is generally present. It should be obvious on examination of the patient that the patient does have COLD prior to the development of these changes.

Interstitial diseases of the lungs may be seen on chest x-ray. Air fluid levels in the retrocardiac area can often be seen in those patients with a hiatal hernia. This may suggest recurrent aspiration as an etiology for reversible obstructive airway disease. After long periods of time, fibrosis can occur in this condition.

Normal x-ray findings do not completely eliminate significant airway disease. Many patients with mild-to-moderate obstructive pulmonary disease, as well as interstitial disease, can have nondiagnostic chest films.[4]

Pulmonary Function Studies

The most sensitive methods for detecting pathologic changes in the respiratory tract are pulmonary function studies. Many times, the history and physical examination, as well as the x-ray examination, are normal even though the pulmonary function studies show rather marked abnormalities. One study demonstrated that 36% of patients with findings of airway obstruction on pulmonary function studies had essentially normal history and physical examination.[5] Often, significant changes of emphysema can be found at autopsy in patients who had not been clinically diagnosed before death. Both the physical and chest x-ray examination often remain normal until late in the disease process.

Patients with pulmonary disease often show deterioration in pulmonary function studies (or improvement in the studies) without significant change in symptomatology. This is well demonstrated in asthmatic patients who are recovering from an acute asthma attack. The patient is usually asymptomatic long before his flow rates return to normal limits. Numerous tests can be used to investigate different aspects of pulmonary physiology in modern pulmonary function laboratories. The patients with complex problems may require certain sophisticated studies to make diagnostic and therapeutic decisions. The majority of patients, however, can be diagnosed by simple spirometry in the physician's office. The patient's vital capacity and expiratory flow rates can be very helpful in determining obstruction to airflow. The spirogram will determine the forced vital capacity (FVC) as well as the forced expiratory volume in various times. The flow expired in the first second (FEV_1) is an important measure of flow in determining obstruction in the airways. Normally, an individual will complete his forced vital capacity manuever in approximately 4 seconds. During the first second, at least 70% of the FVC will be exhaled. In the younger individual, approximately 80% will be exhaled. The ratio of FEV_1/FVC should be greater than 70%. Often, the FEV_1 may be low secondary to a low FVC. The ratio, however, in restrictive disease will remain above 70%.

Of all the pulmonary function tests, the FEV_1 shows the best correlation of clinical severity in patients with COLD.

The forced expiratory flow from 25% to 75% of the FVC (FEF 25–75) may be helpful in determining obstructive pulmonary disease. If the FEV_1 is normal and the FEF 25–75 is decreased, this may give an indication of obstruction primarily in the small airways. This decrease in FEF 25–75 may be reversible with therapy. If the patient's FEV_1 is decreased, generally speaking, the pulmonary function will not return to normal with treatment. Patients with asthma, however, do have reversibility of their airway obstruction, and the FEV_1 may well return to normal limits. Testing

the pulmonary function before and after bronchodilators may show reversibility of the obstructive pattern. In the patient without evidence of airway
obstruction, but in whom the symptomatology is suggestive, studies using
methacholine or histamine challenge may be useful for determining airway
sensitivity to bronchospasm. This may determine the presence of asthma.

Other studies of pulmonary function such as lung volume determinations
and diffusing capacity may be helpful in more fully delineating the physiologic abnormalities in given patients.

Arterial blood gases are also an essential study in evaluating the patient
with respiratory problems. The physiologic mechanisms leading to hypoxia
and hypercapnia may be delineated. The patient at times may have abnormal arterial blood gases while studies of his lung mechanics may not be
significantly abnormal.[3]

Pulmonary Exercise Studies

The reserve capacity of the respiratory system may be markedly decreased before symptomatology develops.[6] A rather large pulmonary reserve is present in the individual with normal lungs. The relationship between clinical symptoms and function derangement can be rather
complicated. Exercise tolerance is a complicated relationship between various components of the body as a whole. An important component of exercise tolerance is the patient's subjective response to the stress of physical
exercise.

Patients often do not perceive a lack of exercise tolerance. The intoler-
ance develops slowly over several years, and the individual gradually reduces his level of exercise and does not become symptomatic until very
late in the disease process.

Because of the above factors, studies during exercise are paramount to
determine the patient's reserve capacity. Exercise testing is also necessary
in determining the interaction between the various systems involved in
oxygen delivery.

Exercise Protocols

There are two types of dynamic exercise employing large muscle groups.
First, in "sprint"-type activity, there is a high-power output over a short
period of time. The second type is steady-state exercise in which the activity lasts over a longer period of time until the patient develops a steady
state regarding oxygen uptake and CO_2 production. Steady state-type exercise is used when estimations of variables requiring several measurements are made.[7]

Several protocols are used in exercise studies. The protocol used must be fitted to the individual being tested and the information sought by the study. Protocols that require high levels of exercise are often not suited to the patient with a disease process, because the patient is often unable to undergo even the first level of exercise. One should devise or utilize a protocol in which the patient is walking or cycling at a comfortable level. A modified Naughton-type protocol has been found useful in a majority of pulmonary patients.[8] In this protocol, the patient is started at 2 mph at a 0 degree grade on the treadmill. The grade is increased by 2.5% every 1 to 2 minutes until the patient reaches a symptom-limited level or until other certain criteria are met for discontinuance of the exercise (Table 4–1).

Certain contraindications to exercise testing must be observed for the safety of the patient. The risks in exercise testing are small but real. It has been estimated that in submaximal testing, the danger of serious arrhythmias or myocardial infarctions is approximately 1:10,000. When one undertakes maximum exercise testing, this danger increases significantly to approximately 1:2,500 in those individuals who have had a previous myocardial infarction. The physician ordering the test has a responsibility for the safety of the patient and must consider the above factors in deciding if the data obtained will be worth the danger involved. Table 4–2 outlines the contraindications to exercise testing.

The indications for an exercise test are varied. They may be divided into indications relative to diagnosis of the etiology of the patient's disease and indications relative to the development of a physiologic profile of the patient (Table 4–3). The physiologic profile allows formation of a rational rehabilitation plan for the patient.

Exercise testing allows measurement of many physiologic variables. The variable measured depends upon the questions asked. Exercise tests measure the response of several systems to the increased demands of oxygen

TABLE 4–1.—INDICATIONS FOR TERMINATING EXERCISE TEST

1. Patient requests discontinuance of test
2. Chest pain of anginal type
3. Subjective sensation of faintness or dizziness
4. Mental confusion
5. Lack of coordination
6. Cyanosis or arterial saturation less than 80% (ear oximetry)
7. Onset of pallor or diaphoresis
8. Frequent premature ventricular beats
9. Paroxysmal ventricular tachycardia
10. Development of atrial arrhythmias absent at rest
11. Ischemia changes on ECG
12. Appearance of bundle branch block or block greater than first degree
13. Fall in systolic pressure below resting value or more than 20 mm Hg drop after exercise rise
14. Systolic blood pressure greater than 280 mm Hg or diastolic pressure greater than 140 mm Hg

TABLE 4–2.—Exercise Testing Contraindications

ABSOLUTE
1. Symptomatic heart failure
2. Unstable angina
3. Myocardial ischemic changes on ECG
4. Acute myocarditis
5. Asthma uncontrolled
6. Hypertension (systolic above 240 mm Hg, diastolic above 120 mm Hg)
7. Febrile illness

RELATIVE
1. Aortic valve disease
2. Recent myocardial infarction (less than 6 weeks previous)
3. Tachycardia (resting above 120 beats per minute)
4. Respiratory failure
5. Uncontrolled diabetes mellitus
6. Electrolyte abnormalities
7. Epilepsy
8. Cerebrovascular disease

supply and CO_2 removal. The following is a list of several questions that may be answered by exercise testing:

1. What is the physiologic reason for certain exercise-induced symptoms such as chest pain or dyspnea?
2. What is the patient's capacity for work?
3. How severely limited is the patient by his disease?
4. Does the patient have more than one diagnosis contributing to the symptomatology, for example, myocardial disease in the patient with obstructive airway disease?
5. What is the effect of therapy on the symptomatology?
6. Are there indications for further investigation of cardiac or pulmonary function?

TABLE 4–3.—Indications for Exercise Testing

DIAGNOSTIC
1. Suspected exercise-induced asthma
2. Suspected coronary insufficiency
3. Suspected exercise-induced arrhythmias
4. Suspected peripheral vascular disease
5. Suspected lack of "physical fitness"
6. Suspected neuromuscular disease

PHYSIOLOGIC PROFILE
1. Known cardiac disease
2. Data for writing exercise prescription
3. Determination of limiting factors in oxygen transport mechanism
4. Determination of occupational disability
5. Classification of impairment

7. Does an organic disease process actually exist that accounts for the patient's symptomatology?
8. What levels of exercise should be prescribed in a rehabilitation program?

Several types of exercise tests may be done to help answer the above questions. These will be reviewed briefly.

Twelve-Minute Walking Test

This is a simple test not requiring elaborate equipment. The patient is asked to walk as far as possible in 12 minutes. The distance is then measured and symptomatology noted.[9] The main questions answered by this test are: (1) How severely limited is the patient by his disease process? (2) What is the effect of therapy on the patient's symptomatology? This test's main attribute is its simplicity and resemblance to the patient's daily activities.

Progressive Standardized Tests

These techniques utilize the treadmill or cycle ergometer. This allows fairly accurate estimation of oxygen consumption during a given work load.[6] Work is increased in increments at 1- to 3-minute time intervals until the patient reaches a symptom-limited work level. The increments usually amount to 100 kilopondmeters/minute, which equals 17 W for a cycle ergometer or an increase of 2.5% grade per minute at a constant

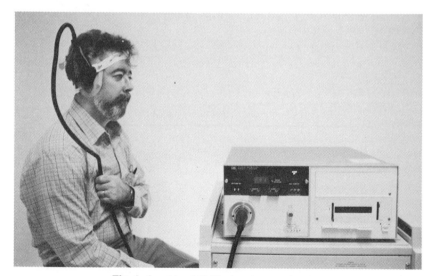

Fig 4–1.—Hewlett-Packard ear oximeter.

speed of 2 mph on the treadmill. Tests may be modified for given patients depending on their tolerance.

During this test, minute ventilation is measured along with its divisions of tidal volume and respiratory frequency. The ECG is also recorded. From this, abnormalities in rhythm, as well as cardiac rate, can be ascertained. Evidence of myocardial ischemia can also be observed.

Analysis of the expired gas for CO_2 and oxygen may also be done. Various parameters may be derived from these results. Ear oximetry should be performed to determine desaturation of hemoglobin during exercise. A drop of more than 2% saturation during exercise is considered significant. The advantage of this type test is that it is within the abilities of most pulmonary or cardiac laboratories, the work load is standardized, and the patient is exercised to the symptom-limited maximum. Much relevant physiologic data that may be clinically useful can be obtained (Figs 4–1 and 4–2).

From this study, information regarding the physiologic reasons for exercise-induced symptoms may be obtained as well as questions regarding the etiology of limitation to exercise. If the tests indicate normal function of the cardiopulmonary system, then reasons for the patient's symptomatology may need to be ruled out by investigating other body systems.

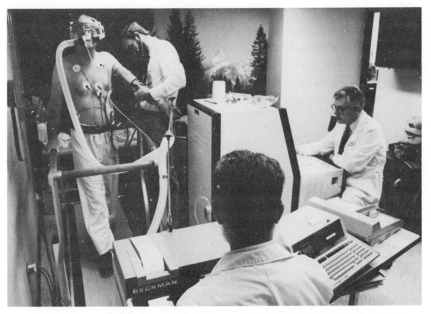

Fig 4–2.—Cardiopulmonary stress testing.

Submaximal Steady-State Studies

Certain derived data require a steady state of oxygen consumption and CO_2 production to be reached. These include V_d/V_t, Qs/Qt (shunt fraction), and cardiac output. These tests are usually done on a cycle ergometer for technical reasons of ease of measurements. The work loads are chosen from the results of the progressive test and related to the patient's maximum work load.[6]

In addition to the measurements made in a progressive test, arterial blood is analyzed for P_{CO_2}, P_{O_2}, pH and lactate. The mixed venous P_{CO_2} is also measured by a rebreathing technique. From these measurements, the cardiac output may be derived. The equations of gas exchange can then be solved (Table 4–4).

These tests are somewhat more difficult to perform and require more sophisticated equipment than the other studies; however, the equipment is available commercially, and the expertise necessary to perform these studies can be developed in most cardiopulmonary laboratories.

The results obtained from this study may be useful in explaining physiologically substandard exercise performance not made clear by the progressive study. If the progressive study has yielded the clinical data sought or the progressive study is normal, little is to be gained from the steady-state study. Changes in gas exchange variables may be useful in following progress of the disease process or results of therapy.

Studies To Determine Exercise-Induced Bronchoconstriction[10]

This study is utilized as a "challenge"-type test to determine the reactivity of the airways. The genesis of bronchial constriction, as a result of running, for example, is most likely airway cooling. In the future, hyperven-

TABLE 4–4.—EQUATIONS OF GAS
EXCHANGE

1. Max. ventilation $= FEV_1 \times 35$
2. $V_d/V_t* = P_{aCO_2} - \dfrac{P_eCO_2}{P_{aCO_2}}$
3. $\dfrac{Qva*}{Qt} = \dfrac{Cc'O_2\dagger - C_aO_2}{Cc'O_2 - C_vO_2}$

*The ratios V_d/V_t and Qva/Q_t are used as indices of pulmonary gas exchange, not as quantitative measurements in exercise. These are clinically useful, although they do represent a simplistic look at complex relationships.
†The $Cc'O_2$ is calculated assuming the end capillary P_{O_2} is equal to the alveolar P_{O_2}.

tilation using cold, dry air may replace exercise as a method of bronchial challenge.[11]

A practical method of performing this study is to measure the FEV_1 prior to exercise and then perform the progressive standardized test. Following the exercise, the FEV_1 is measured at 1, 2, 5, 10, and 15 minutes after exercise. A 20% decrease in the FEV_1 is considered significant. Another method of determining significance is calculation of the bronchial lability index (BLI) of Jones:[7]

$$BLI = \frac{Best\ FEV_1 - Worst\ FEV_1}{Predicted\ FEV_1} \times 100$$

The reason for this calculation being somewhat more discriminating is that often immediately following exercise, transient bronchodilation may occur with an increase in the FEV_1 to above preexercise levels. An increase in the index above 10% indicates significant bronchoconstriction.

Physiologic Picture of the Patient

The objective of obtaining physiologic data on a patient is to develop in the mind's eye a composite picture of the individual both at rest and during exercise. This is of primary importance in order to develop a rational and effective rehabilitation program. The physiologic picture of the patient must also be correlated with the emotional and psychological status of the patient as well as his self-image of the effects that he feels the disease process is having upon his body. One must ultimately approach the individual therapeutically as a whole, and not divide the treatment plan into neat little compartments of physiology, mind, social aspects, etc.

When forming a physiologic picture, one should first give consideration to the mechanics of respiration. The history and physical examination may give clues to the mechanics involved in an individual. Simple spirometry will help in classifying the general pattern of pulmonary mechanics. The FEV_1, peak flow, and FEF 25-75 give an indication of the degree of obstruction to airflow. If decreased, the FVC may suggest the presence of restrictive mechanics. Lung volumes may also be helpful in suggesting the presence and degrees of restrictive mechanics. A decrease in total lung volume indicates restrictive disease. Exercise studies will also give evidence as to the mechanics involved. Normally with exercise, the tidal volume increases first in lower levels of exercise. As the work load increases, the tidal volume increases to a maximum of approximately 60% of the vital capacity. The respiratory rate continues to increase until the product of the tidal volume times the rate equals approximately 35 times the FEV_1.

After mechanics of ventilation are characterized, one's attention may turn to oxygen transport and CO_2 elimination. Because oxygen transport is related to oxygen saturation and cardiac output, one can either measure these variables or estimate them utilizing history and physical data obtained during the exercise study. Gas exchange variables may also be needed at this point to help complete the picture of gas transport and exchange.

It is often useful to draw an actual diagram of the physiologic mechanisms and etiology leading the patient to his present status. This will help in planning the rehabilitation approach.

Once the mind's eye composite physiologic picture of the individual is formed and actually committed to a diagram, it will be much easier to develop a rational rehabilitation program. Techniques may then be determined to utilize in the individual patient to improve his physiologic status. Techniques that will allow the patient to accept those things that cannot be changed and to have a more positive attitude toward his life and his place in society may also be incorporated in the program. Without a full and accurate assessment of the patient as a whole, a rehabilitation program will certainly be less than optimum.

Summary

The various diagnostic techniques for assessing pulmonary dysfunction have a twofold objective. The first objective is to determine the exact etiology of the patient's problem so that appropriate therapeutic measures can be instituted. Secondly, the goal of laboratory testing is prediction of the level at which the patient can perform his daily activities without undue distress or risk to his well-being. It is obvious that the laboratory tests of function may need to be weighed against the independent assessment of the patient's usual activities and level of activity when he was in a healthy state. By utilizing the data obtained during the history and physical examination as well as during various laboratory studies, realistic, goal-oriented pulmonary rehabilitation can be planned and carried out in a meaningful way for the patient.

References

1. Cherniack R.: *Respiration in Health and Disease*, ed. 2. Philadelphia, W.B. Saunders Co., 1972.
2. Godfrey F., Edwards R.H.T., Campbell E.J.M., et al.: Clinical and physiological association of some physical signs observed in patients with chronic airway obstruction. *Thorax* 25:285, 1970.
3. Brashear R.: *Chronic Obstructive Lung Disease*, ed. 1. St. Louis, C.V. Mosby Co., 1978.

4. Alderson P.O., Secker-Walker R.H., Forrest J.V.: Detection of obstructive pulmonary disease: Relative sensitivity of ventilation perfusion studies and chest radiography. *Radiology* 112:643, 1974.
5. Hepper N.G., Hyatt R.E., Fowler W.S.: Detection of chronic obstructive lung disease. *Arch. Environ. Health* 19:806, 1969.
6. Jones N.L.: *Clinical Exercise Testing*, ed. 1. Philadelphia, W.B. Saunders Co., 1975.
7. Clark T.J.H.: *Clinical Investigation of Respiratory Disease*, ed. 1. London, Chapman and Hall Ltd., 1981.
8. Wilson P.K.: *Rehabilitation of the Heart and Lungs*, ed. 1. Fullerton, Calif., Beckman Instruments Inc., 1980.
9. Macgavin C.R., Gupta S.P., McHardy G.H.R.: Twelve minute walking test for assessing disability in chronic bronchitis. *Br. Med. J.* 1:822, 1976.
10. Godfrey S.: Exercise induced asthma: Clinical, physiological and therapeutic implications. *J. Allergy Clin. Immunol.* 56:1, 1975.
11. Strauss R.H.: Enhancement of exercise induced asthma by cold air. *N. Engl. J. Med.* 297:743, 1977.

5 / Hands-on Evaluation

DONALD G. BURNS, D.O.

THE HANDS-ON ASSESSMENT of the patient allows the examiner to arrive at a rational differential diagnosis. Many times, one can diagnose the patient's illness accurately from the interview, or at least arrive at a rational preliminary diagnosis. It is almost always possible to obtain at least a rational differential diagnosis from the hands-on evaluation. By interviewing the patient and doing a complete and painstaking physical examination, not only can one arrive at a differential diagnosis, but one may also appreciate the patient's reaction to his disease process. Confirmation of this diagnosis, as well as refinement of the diagnosis, will usually require more detailed laboratory investigation.

The Patient Interview

In establishing an accurate description of the patient's problem, it is necessary to develop a good rapport. On first meeting the patient, the examiner should explain that he wishes to discuss the details of the illness, and he should approach the individual in a tactful, unhurried, and considerate manner. It is essential that the examiner avoid asking leading questions to which the patient may give the answers that he thinks the examiner desires. In phrasing the questions, the examiner also should use words and phrases that the patient understands. Two common errors in obtaining an accurate description of the patient's problems are that of either talking over the patient's head or talking down to the patient during the interview.

The historical aspect of the patient's problem should be recorded in an orderly, consecutive, and consistent fashion. The interview can be much more efficient if it is conducted in the same manner with each and every patient. This is not to say that one should ask pat questions with each patient. The patient should be allowed to describe his illness as he perceives it. While he is describing his illness, questions may be asked that will help organize the patient's thinking. One should not, however, interrupt the patient to the point that it interferes with his line of thought. Notes should be taken during the interview so that the examiner can later go over the interview results at leisure and put the entire story together in

46

proper perspective. It is often useful for the examiner to have another individual present in the room who is actually taking the notes, so that the patient does not perceive that the examiner is busy writing rather than listening to his story.

One successful method of obtaining the history is first to have the patient describe in depth the onset and course of his present illness. Next, in the pulmonary history, it is important to determine the patient's smoking habits. It is also important to obtain a detailed occupational history of the patient. This should include not only all the jobs that he has had, but also should determine exactly what the patient did in these jobs and for how long. This should start with the first job the patient had and carry through to the present time. One should also ask about the patient's hobbies and any possible exposure to harmful substances. The environmental history is important in determining the patient's previous travel history as well as various places in which the patient has resided.

An accurate description of known allergies should be obtained. A list of medications the patient has taken within the year prior to examination is also useful. A history of past medical and surgical illnesses, as well as any complications that have occurred with these, is mandatory. A review of other bodily systems then should be carried out to determine symptoms in systems other than the respiratory system. A family history regarding infectious diseases, as well as diseases that may have genetic predisposition, is also important. It is helpful to record in an orderly manner the patient's various cardinal respiratory symptoms, including dyspnea, cough, wheeze, chest pain, and hemoptysis. Some useful guidelines for obtaining a good pulmonary history follow.

PRESENTING COMPLAINTS.—The presenting complaints are what the patient perceives as the most prominent symptoms. These are the ones that prompted him to obtain medical care and should be recorded in order of the patient's perceived order of importance. It is often best to ask the patient when he last felt well and then note each symptom in the order of its onset. This information can help the examiner ascertain whether he is dealing with an acute illness or possibly a subacute or chronic illness. The examiner must also determine whether the illness has remained stationary or progressed in severity. If the illness has been complicated by any acute exacerbations, this should be established.

CARDINAL SYMPTOMS.—The patient should be asked specifically regarding the symptoms of dyspnea, cough, hemoptysis, wheezing, and chest pain. Each of these symptoms should be detailed regarding onset as well as severity and chronicity. Factors that modify these symptoms, either causing an exacerbation or relief, should be determined and recorded.

SMOKING HISTORY.—A history of the patient's smoking habits is essential and should include the age at which the patient began smoking as well as the current daily consumption of cigarettes, cigars, or pipe tobacco. The concept of number of packs smoked per day times the years smoked (pack years) is useful. If the patient has stopped smoking, the date should be recorded and the reasons noted. Cigarette smoking is linked to the development of bronchogenic carcinoma and is particularly important in the pathogenesis of chronic bronchitis as well as emphysema.

FAMILY HISTORY.—All serious illnesses that have affected any member of the patient's immediate family should be recorded as well as the cause of death and age at death of any deceased relative. It is important to attempt to determine diseases that have hereditary predisposition such as cystic fibrosis or asthma. It is essential to obtain the family history of infectious illnesses such as tuberculosis.

ENVIRONMENTAL HISTORY.—The patient's environment, as well as his background and living habits, may have a bearing on the development of his illness. The various areas in which the patient has lived or traveled should be listed together with the amount of time spent in each area. Certain areas are notorious for endemic diseases. Histoplasmosis is endemic in the valleys of the Ohio, St. Lawrence, and Mississippi rivers; coccidiomycosis is found in the arid deserts of Southern California, Arizona, Mexico, West Texas, and New Mexico. The incidence of schistosomiasis is high in Puerto Rico and Egypt. The patient's socioeconomic status and that of his parents should also be elicited, because certain ethnic groups have higher susceptibility to certain diseases.

OCCUPATIONAL HISTORY.—A complete and detailed occupational history is important. The duration of each term of employment and the exact job that the patient performed should be listed. Occupations involving exposure to high levels of dust fumes or smoke may lead to the development of chronic bronchitis. Those involved in manufacturing with beryllium may develop berylliosis; inhalation of asbestos fibers predisposes to asbestosis, fibrosis, bronchogenic carcinoma, and mesothelioma.

PERSONAL HISTORY.—The patient's habits may influence his ability to resist disease, and these should be elicited. Worries or anxieties may increase susceptibility to disease. The nutritional status of the patient may also influence the immunologic state and susceptibility to certain diseases. A history of alcohol intake may be helpful in determining the patient's resistance to various diseases, especially those of infectious origin. Does the patient have close contact with pets or flowers? Attacks of bronchial asthma may be precipitated by exposure to the dander of dogs, cats, or horses as well as pollens of various plants. Interstitial pneumonitis may be associated with diseased birds.

PAST MEDICAL ILLNESSES.—The past illnesses, including infectious diseases of childhood, should be recorded. A history of infantile eczema, atopic dermatitis, or allergic rhinitis should be recorded. Measles, adenoviral infections, or pertussis in childhood, especially if prolonged or complicated by pneumonia, may predispose the individual to bronchiectasis.

PAST SURGICAL ILLNESSES.—Pulmonary abscesses may follow dental extractions, upper respiratory tract surgery, or aspiration of foreign bodies. Previous injuries or surgery on the chest may be the cause of fibrothorax or cardiorespiratory insufficiency.

Review of Systems

NERVOUS SYSTEM.—Cerebral abscess secondary to bronchiectasis may cause severe intractable throbbing headaches as well as paresis, drowsiness, diplopia, disorientation, confusion, and syncopal attacks. Many of these symptoms may also be caused by hypoxia and hypercarbia. Occasionally, patients with severe chronic respiratory insufficiency are admitted to neurologic wards because of suspicion of an expanding intracerebral lesion.

CARDIOVASCULAR SYSTEM.—The cardiovascular system closely intertwines with the pulmonary system. Cough and dyspnea are symptoms of cardiac disease as well as pulmonary disease. Orthopnea and an increase in the number of pillows used at night may be suggestive of the onset of left ventricular failure. A recent attack of substernal chest pain followed by dyspnea may suggest a myocardial infarction and congestive heart failure.

Increasing breathlessness and ankle swelling often point to the development of right-sided heart failure secondary to pulmonary disease. An attack of pleuritic-type chest pain in the patient with heart failure may be compatible with a pulmonary embolus.

GASTROINTESTINAL SYSTEM.—Dysphagia may be secondary to malignant processes in the esophagus or stricture of the esophagus, which may lead to aspiration. Aspiration may also occur secondary to a hiatal hernia or achalasia of the esophageal sphincter. Anorexia and vague gastrointestinal complaints are often associated with active pulmonary tuberculosis or chronic bronchopulmonary disease. Postprandial epigastric pain relieved by the ingestion of food and alkali suggest peptic ulceration, which is a common occurrence in association with chronic respiratory disease. Chronic diarrhea may indicate the development of amyloidosis in a patient who is suffering from a suppurative pulmonary disease such as tuberculosis.

GENITOURINARY SYSTEM.—Hematuria, along with frequency and dysuria, may possibly be secondary to renal tuberculosis. Hematuria can also be produced by renal carcinoma. Painful testicles may indicate either tuberculosis or malignant involvement. Amenorrhea often accompanies pulmonary tuberculosis.

METABOLIC SYSTEM.—Weight loss, along with general malaise and fatigue, is often present in chronic respiratory disease. Considerable weight loss may occur in active tuberculosis or malignancy, and excessive weight gain may be associated with sleep apnea syndromes as well as hypertension.

LOCOMOTOR SYSTEMS.—If clubbing of the fingers is noted in the patient, the time of onset should be elicited. Recent onset often suggests a malignancy. Pain or tenderness to palpation in the lower parts of the forearm or legs may be caused by hypertrophic pulmonary osteoarthropathy. A flapping tremor of the hands may be seen in severe CO_2 retention and acidemia. A fine tremor may indicate hyperthyroidism and can be the cause of dyspnea. Painful, tender, purplish discolorations of erythema nodosum often occur over the extensor surfaces of the legs and may be due to sarcoidosis or tuberculosis. The onset of weakness in specific groups of muscles may be suggestive of myopathy associated with pulmonary malignancy or neuromuscular disease.

MEDICATIONS.—It is important to know the medications that the patient has been taking over the recent past. Many times, the patient's symptoms are a direct result of the side effects caused by drugs. A general summary of the portions of the history usually obtained is listed in Table 5–1.

Physical Examination

After obtaining a comprehensive history, the examiner is often able to synthesize the pertinent aspects of the history into various patterns, thereby formulating a differential diagnosis. The differential diagnosis may then be strengthened and perhaps confirmed by the physical examination. A mastery of the technique of physical examination is paramount in arriving at a correct diagnosis.

TABLE 5–1.—SUMMARY OF SECTIONS
OF HISTORY

1. Presenting complaints
2. Cardinal respiratory symptoms
3. Smoking history
4. Occupational history
5. Travel and environmental history
6. Family history
7. Social history
8. Present medications
9. Allergies
10. Past medical history
11. Past surgical history
12. Review of systems

Becoming proficient in the physical examination can only be obtained by repeated examination of healthy individuals. This is essential so that one can recognize even minimal abnormalities. Examination of the nonrespiratory system is also important. A physical examination should be carried out in a systematic manner in every patient so that no abnormalities are overlooked.

A detailed description of the examination of the respiratory system is presented in the following discussion. The methods of examination of the remaining systems will not be discussed. Only those findings that may be helpful in assessing the findings in the respiratory system will be discussed.

OBSERVATION.—Observation of the patient is the initial phase of the physical examination. This should be meticulously conducted to elicit signs of disease. The observation of the patient actually begins during the interview. Much is learned from observation and is aquired subconsciously. For example, most examiners can make an accurate guess of the patient's age without consciously doing so. Yet, they are usually unable to describe the physical evidence upon which this judgment is based. Often, looking at the patient gives indication whether they are well or ill. The actual evidence upon which this judgment is based is very difficult to describe; often it is a combination of experience coupled with empiric judgment.

FACE AND HEAD.—Enumeration of all the factors that may be detected from an even casual glance at the patient's face is not possible, but one can generally determine the degree of distress the patient is experiencing. It is possible from the patient's facial expression to estimate the temperament and mood of the patient and sometimes to recognize impaired mental capacity. Other findings such as the presence of respiratory distress, cyanosis, or plethora may be evident. The examiner should also look for evidence of edema, venous dilatation, emaciation, or obesity.

Respiratory distress is particularly important to note and observe, considering whether it is largely inspiratory or expiratory in nature. Obvious use of the accessory muscles of respiration is easily determined. The rate of respiration, as well as the tidal volume, also can be estimated. The general position the patient assumes should be observed. In severe dyspnea, the patient will assume a characteristic posture with the trunk bent forward and the hands on the thighs.

Breathing patterns should be observed regarding the depth as well as the frequency of respiration. Whether the respirations are regular or irregular should be noted. Localizing neurologic signs are suggestive of cerebral metastasis or perhaps of cerebral abscess secondary to bronchiectasis. Confusion may be observed in the patient who has severe hypoxia or hypercarbia.

EYES.—Fundoscopic examination often reveals engorged vessels during acute respiratory failure. Miliary tuberculosis may produce small, round miliary nodules seen on funduscopic examination. The pupils also can be affected by respiratory distress. Irritation of the cervical sympathetic ganglia by disease in the apex of the lung causes dilatation of the pupil on the side of the lesion. This is often seen in Pancoast's tumor. Metastatic lymph nodes may cause dilatation of the pupil on the side of metastasis. With progression of the disease, the sympathetic ganglia may become paralyzed and the affected pupil constricted. There may be absence of sweating on the affected side of the face and the development of a so-called Horner's syndrome.

NECK.—Engorgement of the veins in the neck in the patient whose head is elevated at an angle of 45 degrees is abnormal and indicates that the venous pressure is elevated. Bilateral jugular venous distention is generally due to congestive heart failure, although it is possible that it is increased secondary to obstruction of the superior vena cava. Distention of the jugular veins during expiration is not unusual in patients suffering from severe obstructive lung disease. This is due to an increase in intrathoracic pressure during the expiratory process.

Cervical lymphadenopathy is due to numerous conditions, including sarcoidosis, malignancy, and mononucleosis. One should look for scars on the neck that may be the result of tuberculous adenitis. Palpation of the neck is used in determining the various masses that may not have been obvious on observation. Palpation of the neck should be carried out with the fingertips and using gentle pressure, first examining the posterior and then the anterior triangles of the neck as well as the submental areas. The supraclavicular areas of the neck should also be palpated. Nodes palpated in this area may be the result of bronchogenic carcinoma.

HANDS.—Clubbing of the fingers is an important finding in respiratory disease. On examination, the profile of the terminal phalanx of the finger, the angle between the proximal end of the nail and the soft tissues covering its root, is approximately 160 degrees. The earliest sign of clubbing is hypertrophy of the soft tissue to the extent that this base angle is obliterated and becomes 180 degrees or greater. Palpation of this area may also detect softness secondary to hypertrophy of the tissue. The index finger and the thumb are usually the first affected by clubbing, the other fingers becoming involved as the condition progresses. Generally, the clubbing is bilateral.[3]

Obliteration of the base angle is a primary feature throughout the progress of clubbing. As the clubbing becomes more severe, the skin overlying the nail bed becomes stretched and loses its normal wrinkles so that it looks quite shiny. The nail then becomes gradually thickened and curved.

The pulp of the terminal phalanx gradually becomes bulbous in appearance. In advanced clubbing, the nail is thickened, ridged, and curved longitudinally as well as transversely. The distal end of the nail overrides the end of the finger so that it resembles a beak. On palpation of the nail, it is easily compressed and often gives the impression of lying on a bed of fluid.

The hallmark of clubbing is the base angle that is more than 160 degrees.[1] Curved nails are occasionally found in healthy people and may easily be confused with clubbing.

Hypertrophic pulmonary osteoarthropathy, the last stage in the progression of digital clubbing, is characterized by painful, tender thickening of both the wrists and ankles in association with digital clubbing. There are inflammatory changes in the subcutaneous tissues, the capsule, and the synovial membrane of the ankle and wrist joints as well as periostitis of the lower ends of the long bones of the arms and legs. Presence of hypertrophic pulmonary osteoarthropathy is suggestive of pulmonary malignancy.

THE UPPER RESPIRATORY TRACT.—Diseases that affect the lower respiratory tract often also affect the upper respiratory tract.

Patency of the nasal passages may be tested by having the patient sniff through each nostril while occluding the opposite nostril. One may also observe the nasal passages with an otoscope. Nasal polyps may be obvious and are associated with allergy. Allergic nasal membranes appear pale and swollen, and a thin, watery discharge is often present. If infection is present, thick yellow or green exudate may be seen.

Examination of the mouth may be helpful. Halitosis may result from improper hygiene; however, it may also be present from infected tonsils or sinuses. Septic diseases of the lungs such as abscess can cause bad breath. The teeth and gums should be examined for poor dental care, because this may be a factor in the development of pulmonary abscesses. The larynx should also be examined, either by indirect means with a mirror or by direct examination. By the indirect method, the patient's tongue is held out with gauze, and a warmed laryngeal mirror is placed against the soft palate in front of the uvula. With a light from either a head mirror or a head light, the epiglottis, arytenoid regions, and vocal cords may be viewed. It is important to examine the vocal cords during phonation to determine the presence of unilateral vocal cord paralysis. One should also look for laryngeal obstruction by polyps or tumor.

EXAMINATION OF THE CHEST.—Before an adequate and precise examination can be made, there must be a clear mental picture of the lobes or segments being examined. Because of this, the surface anatomy of the chest will be reviewed. Figures 5–1, 5–2, and 5–3 will aid the reader as he reads the text portion.

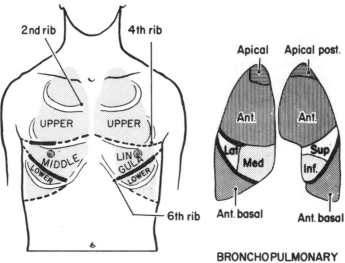

SURFACE MARKINGS

BRONCHOPULMONARY SEGMENTS

Fig 5–1.—Surface markings of the lungs (anterior aspect) and underlying bronchopulmonary segments. (From Cherniack R.: *Respiration in Health and Disease,* ed. 2. Philadelphia, W.B. Saunders Co., 1972. Used by permission.)

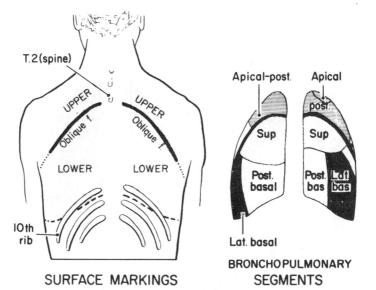

SURFACE MARKINGS

BRONCHOPULMONARY SEGMENTS

Fig 5–2.—Surface markings of the lungs (posterior aspect) and underlying bronchopulmonary segments. (From Cherniack R.: *Respiration in Health and Disease,* ed. 2. Philadelphia, W.B. Saunders Co., 1972. Used by permission.)

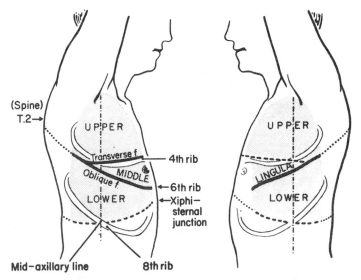

Fig 5–3.—Surface markings of the lungs (lateral aspect). (From Cherniack R.: *Respiration in Health and Disease,* ed. 2. Philadelphia, W.B. Saunders Co., 1972. Used by permission.)

The sternal angle and the spinous processes of the dorsal vertebra enable the examiner to orient himself regarding the position of the underlying chest content. In the erect subject with head bent slightly forward, the first thoracic spine is the lower of two prominent projections at the junction of the neck and thorax. The upper projection is the spinous process of the seventh cervical vertebra. The kidney angle is at the junction of the posterior end of the costal margin and the sacrospinal muscle. This is at the level of the 12th dorsal vertebra.

The sternal angle is at the level of bifurcation of the trachea. This is also the upper limit of the atria of the heart as well as the approximate upper level at which the lungs meet anteriorly. The sternal angle is also a landmark for identification of the ribs. The second costal cartilage articulates with the sternum at the sternal angle, and from this knowledge, other ribs, cartilages, and interspaces may be identified by palpation.

Certain lines are used to demarcate various areas of the chest wall. The midclavicular line runs vertically downward from the middle of the clavicles to the lower costal margin anteriorly. The midscapular posterior line runs vertically downward from the middle of the inferior angle of the scapula to the kidney angle. The anterior lateral axillary line runs vertically downward from the origin of the anterior axillary fold; the posterior axillary line runs downward from the border of the posterior axillary fold. The mid-axillary line runs vertically downward over the lateral aspect of the chest from the middle of the apex of the axillae to the lower costal margin, midway between the anterior and posterior axillary lines.

Surface markings.—Both lungs are closely covered in the apices by the pleurae and lie in the root of the neck, starting at the lower end of the sternoclavicular junction and curving upward to approximately 2.5 cm above the clavicle. They then descend to the lower end of the clavicle at the junction of its lateral and middle thirds. The anterior border of the pleural space on the right is indicated by a line drawn from the sternoclavicular joint to the center of the sternal angle. The line then turns downward to the xiphosternal joint. The surface markings at the anterior border of the right lung correspond almost exactly to that of the right pleura. The anterior border of the left pleural space may be indicated by a line drawn from the left sternoclavicular joint to the center of the sternoangle and then vertically downward to the level of the fourth costal cartilage. The line then turns laterally to the left border of the sternum and vertically to the seventh costal cartilage. The anterior border of the left lung occupies essentially the same position inside the pleura until the fourth left costal cartilage is reached. The lung then turns laterally along the fourth coastal cartilage to a point approximately 3 cm lateral to the left sternal border. The line then turns downward and ends at the sixth costal cartilage approximately 2.5 cm from the border of the sternum.

Inferiorly, the borders of both pleural spaces correspond to a line starting at the lower ends of the anterior margins, then running backward and crossing the sixth ribs at the midclavicular line, the eighth ribs in the midaxillary line, and the 12th ribs at the midscapular line. The inferior borders then end approximately 2.5 cm lateral to the 12th thoracic spine. The inferior borders of both lungs correspond to those of the pleura and the anterior portion crossing the midclavicular and midaxillary line at the sixth and eighth ribs respectively. Thereafter, they cross the midscapular line at the tenth rib posteriorly and at the level of the tenth thoracic spine. The posterior borders of the pleura and lungs run parallel to each other, that of the lung being just lateral to the pleural border.

The major fissures in both lungs separate the upper and lower lobes. The course of these may be illustrated on the surface of the chest wall by a line starting at the second thoracic spine posteriorly and running obliquely downward curving down the chest wall. It crosses the midaxillary line at the fifth rib and ends anteriorly at the inferior border of the sixth costal cartilage midway between the midsternal and midclavicular lines. With the patient standing erect and placing his hands behind his neck, the position of the scapula is such that the vertebral borders correspond to the posterior parts of the oblique fissures. The minor fissure separates the middle lobe from the upper lobe on the right. The transverse fissure may be outlined on the chest wall, but starts at the anterior border of the lung at the level of the third or fourth intercostal space. It then passes laterally in a slightly upward direction, ending at the point where the oblique fissure crosses the midaxillary line.

The bronchopulmonary segments lie within the confines of the boundaries of the lobes. The anterior segment in both upper lobes lies in an area between the transverse fissure, as described above, and the clavicles. The apical segment of the right upper lobe lies within an area above the clavicle anteriorly and a small area posterior in the apex of the lung. The remainder of the posterior aspect of the right upper lobe is occupied by the posterior segment. The apical posterior segment of the left upper lobe lies in an area similar to that of the apical and posterior segments of the right upper lobe. The right middle lobe is divided into the medial and lateral segments. The medial segments occupy the anterior portion of the chest between the areas of the third interspace and the major fissure anteriorly. The lateral segment occupies the remaining portion of the middle lobe area in the anterior portion of the axillae. On the left side, the lingular portion of the left upper lobe occupies an area of the left side corresponding to that of the right middle lobe on the right side. The lingular portion is divided into two segments, the superior and inferior. The lingular area is divided roughly in half, with the upper portion occupied by the superior segment and the lower portion occupied by the inferior segment.

The surface anatomy of the two lower lobes is very similiar. The superior segment occupies the upper part of the posterior aspect of the lower lobe, its upper border being the major fissure and its lower boundary corresponding to the spinous process of the seventh dorsal vertebra. The remainder of the posterior aspect of the lower lobe area is occupied by the posterior basilar segment. The axillary aspect of the lower lobe is occupied by the lateral basilar segment. The anterior basilar segment lies under the anterior chest wall in the lower lobe. The medial basal segment lies next to the mediastinum and has no comparable area over the surface of the chest wall.[1]

Palpation.—The position of the mediastinum can be determined by palpation of two areas. Palpation of the position of the trachea and the cardiac impulse can give a good indication of the mediastinal position. The trachea is normally in the midline position, except on occasion in elderly persons in whom it may be shifted to the right normally because of pressure by an atheromatous ascending aorta. In general, a shift of the trachea from its midline position is indicative of some intrathoracic disease.

The position of the trachea may best be determined while the patient is either in a sitting position or recumbent in bed with the neck slightly flexed. The sternocleidomastoid muscles must be relaxed and the chin in the midline position. The lowest portion of the trachea just before it enters the thoracic inlet is the most mobile portion of the trachea and is the portion in which the examiner is most interested. The tip of the examiner's fully extended index finger is inserted into the suprasternal notch and is gently pressed backward toward the cervical spine, first on one side and then the other. If the trachea is in a normal midline position, the examining finger will strike only soft tissue on both sides of the trachea. If the trachea is deviated from this position, the examining finger will encounter the cartilaginous rings of the trachea of the side to which the mediastinum is shifted.

The apical impulse of the heart is best palpated with the palm of the hand, which is moved from the midaxillary line toward the sternum until the impulse is felt. Using the tips of the fingers, the most lateral systolic impact may be defined. At times in obese subjects or those suffering from COLD, this is difficult or impossible to feel. With the hand in the inframammary region, the intensity of the cardiac impulse should be noted. A very localized systolic thrust is felt normally; however, with left ventricular hypertrophy, a heave is imparted to the ribs. A rocking-type motion is noted in right ventricular hypertrophy, and the thrust is felt just to the left of the sternum with simultaneous retraction over the apex of the left ventricle. If this apical impulse is more than 8 cm from the midsternal line, at the fifth left interspace, the heart is either displaced or hypertrophied. If the trachea is in the midline and the apical impulse is shifted laterally, then left ventricular hypertrophy is present. The source of chest wall pain may require a careful and systematic palpation of the chest wall for tender areas. One should first start away from the painful area, following along the course of the ribs and intercostal spaces. At times, a small peripheral pulmonary embolus may cause acute pleuritis associated with exquisite tenderness in the intercostal space over this area.

Movement of the chest wall may be determined by palpation of the chest. Reduced inflation of a portion of the lung may be reflected by diminished movement of the overlying area of the chest wall. The chest wall movement may be assessed by stretching the skin of the chest wall toward the middle of the chest with the examiner's hands while the patient is breathing quietly. Then one allows the hands to follow the chest wall movement while the patient breaths deeply. The elbows and shoulders of the examiner should be maintained in a relaxed state and only the wrists used to apply pressure on the chest wall. This allows the shoulders to act as a fulcrum, which will exaggerate the movement of the hands. If both areas of the lungs are distending normally, the hands will move an equal distance away from each other with inspiration. It is the comparison of the two sides that is important rather than the extent of the movement.

Movement of the upper lobes is determined by placing the hands over the first four ribs anteriorly with the fingers extending and overlying the trapezius muscle. The skin is then stretched by dragging the palms of the hands downward until the palms lie firmly over the infraclavicular areas while the fingers remain over the supraclavicular areas. Keeping the thumbs fully extended, the skin is pulled medially toward the sternum until the tips of both thumbs meet at the midsternal line. The movement of the hands and thumbs are observed while the patient inspires deeply.

The middle lobe of the right lung and the lingular areas of the left upper lobe underly the corresponding fifth and sixth ribs. On inspiration, this portion of the chest wall moves in both an anterior-posterior and a lateral direction. Largely, the lateral expansion of these ribs is tested. This is done while the patient faces the examiner and the outstretched fingers of both hands are placed over the posterior axillary folds high up in the axillae with the palms flat against the anterior chest wall. The skin is then pulled medially until the outstretched thumbs meet at the midsternal line. Once again, the movement of the hands and thumbs are observed while the patient inspires deeply.

Movement of the lower lobes is determined with the patient sitting with his back to the examiner. These lobes underly the corresponding seventh to tenth ribs, and inspiratory expansion of this part of the chest takes wholly in a lateral direction. The examiner places both his hands high up on the axillae with the outstretched fingers overlying the anterior axillary folds. Both hands are then drawn medially, stretching the underlying skin until the outstretched thumbs meet in the midline over the spinous processes. The movement of the hands and thumbs are then observed while the patient inspires deeply. The lower lobes also expand vertically because of the diaphragmatic motion. To determine this motion, the examiner stands beside the supine patient and places his hands lightly over the anterior lower chest wall while both thumbs overlie the respective costal margins. The thumbs meet over the xiphoid processes. When the patient breathes deeply, the thumbs should move away from each other for an equal distance if the dome shape of the diaphragm is not altered. If the diaphragms are flat, as occurs in COLD, the costal margins will move inward instead of outward.[3] This finding is described as Hoover's sign.

Vocal fremitus is produced by vibrations conducted through the tracheobronchial tree and lung parenchyma during phonation. This may be detected by listening with a stethoscope. By placing the side of the hand over the chest wall, the vibrations may be felt. This is traditionally called "tactile fremitus." Using the side of the hand, the examiner can detect vibrations while the patient slowly repeats a combination of words such as "ninety-nine, ninety-nine." Often, there is a marked difference either in an increased or decreased intensity of vibrations when the side of the hand reaches an area of disease. This may be difficult to palpate if the patient is quite obese or in individuals who have voices that are less resonant. Tactile fremitus is increased in intensity whenever the density of the underlying lung parenchyma is increased in changes such as consolidation. The underlying bronchi must be patent for this vibration to reach the examining hand. Tactile fremitus is diminished if there is fluid or air in the pleural space or when obstruction in the bronchus has led to atelectasis.

Percussion.—Percussion of the chest is carried out to determine if there is change in the density of the underlying areas of the lung pleura or pleural space. Indirect percussion is the most common technique. Here the left middle finger is placed lightly on the chest wall while the terminal phalanx is applied with very little pressure. The other four fingers are raised slightly so that damping of the percussion note does not take place. The middle finger of the right hand is then brought sharply at a right angle to tap the terminal phalanx pleximeter finger in a rapid staccato manner. The blows should be short, sharp, and light, with instantaneous recoil of the finger. If the percussion is too forceful, large areas of the chest wall will be made to vibrate so that the underlying pulmonary lesion may be missed. If the lesion is small and more than approximately 5 cm below the chest wall, it may not be detected.

Well-aerated lung parenchyma produces a low-pitched, resonant sound, whereas the sound that is higher in pitch with a dull note implies that the amount of solid tissue beneath the percussing finger is increased. This may be due to atelectasis, fibrosis, or consolidation as well as fluid in the pleural space.

It is best to percuss over healthy lung first and then move slowly to the area of suspected pathology. The borders of an abnormal area of percussion should be outlined by percussing from above and below as well as from each side. To be certain that the pitch is truly altered, comparison of the opposite side should be carried out. Small collections of fluid in the pleural space may be difficult to differentiate from that of an elevated diaphragm. Percussing while having the patient inspire deeply may show that the upper limit of dullness moves downward and would suggest an elevated diaphragm.

Auscultation.—Normal breath sounds can be appreciated by placing the stethoscope over the axillary region with the patient breathing normally. Here it is noted that the inspiratory phase is easily heard and the expiratory phase is considerably fainter, approximating only one third the length of the inspiratory phase. This is the type of breath sound that should normally be heard over the entire chest. In the supraclavicular area on the right, however, the bronchovesicular-type sound is heard because of the fact that the bronchi lie closer to the chest wall in this area.

Appreciation of bronchovesicular breath sounds may be heard by listening over the right supraclavicular area. Here the inspiration is heard clearly; however, the expiratory phase of breath sounds is much louder and may be heard in its entirety.

Bronchial breath sounds can be appreciated by listening over one's own trachea at the upper portion of the sternum where lung tissue does not lie between the airway and the stethoscope. In bronchial breath sounds, the inspiratory and expiratory notes are equal in pitch and are separated by a silent interval. This breath sound is called "bronchial." It means that a disease process has become rather extensive and there is considerable loss of air-containing alveoli. It also indicates patent bronchi are surrounded by solid lung tissue. The feature that distinguishes bronchial breath sounds from bronchovesicular sounds is that in the former the inspiratory phase runs directly into the expiratory phase. In bronchial breath sounds, however, there is a silent interval between end-inspiration and beginning expiration.

Whispering pectoriloquy may be useful in determining small areas of consolidation. Here the patient whispers a combination of words such as "ninety-nine." If the whispered words cannot be heard, the situation is normal. When vibrations are transmitted to the chest wall, the underlying tissue is consolidated.

Egophony is an alteration in the quality of the sound heard when the patient speaks. Here the patient does not whisper, but speaks in a normal tone of voice. The words come through loudly and with great clarity with a bleating quality if consolidation is present under the stethoscope.

The presence of adventitious sounds indicate that some type of pathologic process has developed in the affected area.

Wheezes are prolonged musical or whistling notes produced within the lumen of the bronchial tree. This is indicative of increased turbulence within the airways. Wheezing becomes more pronounced during the expiratory phase of ventilation and is made more noticeable by forced expiration. Low-pitched quality wheezes are usually produced in the larger bronchi, whereas high-pitched wheezes are from the smaller bronchi. At times, these may be best heard by listening over the open mouth while the patient expires his air forcibly. If the wheeze is heard in one portion of the chest wall, it may signify a localized partial obstruction due to tumor or possibly foreign objects.

Crackles are moist, short, disconnected, bubbling-type sounds heard most readily during inspiration. Low-pitched crackles heard in the initial third of the respiratory phase suggest that secretions are present in the larger bronchi, whereas high-pitched crackles heard during the terminal third of inspiration suggest that lung parenchyma may be involved.[2]

A pleural friction rub is a leathery-type sound heard at the end of inspiration and the beginning of expiration. The friction rub is diagnostic of pleural irritation. Since the excursion of the pleural surfaces is greater over the lower lobes than the upper, friction rubs are most frquently detected in the lower-lobe areas.

Auscultation of the heart sounds may be helpful in determining signs of pulmonary heart disease. Auscultation of the intensity of the second pulmonic heart sound should be noted; an increase in this intensity may suggest that pulmonary hypertension is present. The pulmonic second sound is normally split and is accentuated during inspiration. This is caused by a prolongation of the right ventricular systole secondary to increased filling of the right ventricle during inspiration. If this split does not widen during inspiration, it is a further sign of the presence of pulmonary hypertension. A prolonged split of the second pulmonic sound during inspiration may be caused, however, by a delay in closure of the pulmonic valve, which may be secondary to a bundle branch block or a possible mild pulmonary stenosis. A high-pitched systolic ejection click in the pulmonic area may also be indicative of pulmonary hypertension. This occurs during systole just after opening of the pulmonic valve at the end of the period of isometric contraction. This is usually found in patients with large left-to-right shunts, mild pulmonary stenosis, or dilatation of the pulmonary artery.

Assessment of the degree of pulmonary obstruction may also be determined by listening over the chest while the patient takes a full inspiration and attempts a complete expiratory maneuver. The length of time taken for the patient to empty his lungs forcibly should be noted. If this is more than approximately 5 seconds, it gives a good indication for the presence of a rather severe obstruction to airflow.

OTHER ASPECTS OF THE GENERAL PHYSICAL EXAMINATION.—The abdomen should be palpated to determine whether abnormal masses or enlargement of the liver or spleen is present. Metastatic infiltration of the liver from a bronchogenic carcinoma or one of the lymphomas may cause abnormalities in the abdomen. Rectal examination should be carried out to determine if carcinoma of the rectum is present. The prostate gland should also be examined at this time for changes suggesting malignant processes that may be the source of pulmonary metastasis.

The external genitalia should be examined for scars. A primary chancre caused by syphilis may suggest the possibility of an aortic aneurysm. Tuberculosis epididymitis may cause suspicion of an active pulmonary tuberculosis.

TABLE 5–2.—SUMMARY OF SECTIONS OF PHYSICAL EXAMINATION

	OBSERVATION	PALPATION	AUSCULTATION	PERCUSSION
General	+*	–†	–	–
Head	+	+	–	–
Neck	+	+	+	–
Chest	+	+	+	+
Abdomen	+	+	+	+
Extremities	+	+	–	–

*Performed.
†Not performed.

The skin should be examined for pallor suggesting anemia. The presence of cyanosis should be noted as well as pigmentation of the skin creases suggesting Addison's disease. Atopic dermatitis or urticaria may be present as well as erythema nodosum. This may be suggestive of tuberculosis, sarcoidosis, or one of the deep fungal infections. Chronic infiltration of the skin may also occur with sarcoidosis as well as with histiocytosis X. Table 5–2 summarizes the physical examination process.

Summary

Abnormal findings elicited during the interview and physical examination of the patient may indicate the presence of certain categories of disease as well as their approximate location. By considering historical information along with the physical examination, one may generally arrive at an accurate presumptive clinical diagnosis. This diagnosis should be supplemented by an assessment of the effect of the disease on pulmonary function both at rest and during exercise.

References

1. Brashear R.E.: *Chronic Obstructive Lung Disease,* ed. 1. St. Louis, C.V. Mosby Co., 1978.
2. Cherniack R.M.: *Respiration in Health and Disease,* ed. 2. Philadelphia, W.B. Saunders Co., 1972.
3. Forgoes P.: Crackles and wheezes. *Lancet* ii:203, 1967.

6 / Pulmonary Rehabilitation Techniques

JERRY A. O'RYAN, B.S., R.R.T.

CHAPTERS 2 THROUGH 5 discussed the preliminary steps required prior to starting a patient in a pulmonary rehabilitation program. This chapter will discuss many of the actual techniques used in the breathing training and exercise of the chronic obstructive lung-diseased COLD patient. It is at this point that the patient ceases merely being a passive subject of study, prodded and tested, and starts being an active participant in his care.

Principles of Breathing Training and Exercise

Breathing training (or *retraining*) must occur before the patient attempts to exercise. Breathing training consists of the fundamental education and low-level physical activities the patient needs to master before he attempts the more conventional exercises such as walking, climbing stairs, cycling, and treadmill workouts. These preliminary activities will serve to reeducate the patient in proper breathing techniques, the desired outcome being a patient with improved ventilatory efficiency and increased exercise tolerance relative to his disease state.

For a point of reference and degree, the concepts of breathing training and exercise are defined as follows:

1. *Breathing training* consists of the initial and ongoing verbal and physical (hands-on) coaching by the therapist. It will include the teaching of diaphragmatic-pursed lip breathing (D-PLB) as well as useful range of motion (ROM) activities that can be modified and incorporated into the everyday movements required of the patient as he performs domestic or occupational functions. Other elements of breathing training include the teaching of basic pathophysiology regarding lung disease, use of audiovisual aids to punctuate and heighten the learning process, and counseling as needed.

2. The concept of *exercise* is used primarily in the conventional sense and would include the aforementioned walking, stair-climbing, cycling, and treadmill activities. Exercise is a goal-oriented activity, the goals being (1) an increase in work capacity, (2) an increase in maximum oxygen uptake,

(3) an increase in endurance, and (4) acquiring a level of homeostasis greater than the pretraining period.

Task-Specific Concept

The idea of the *task-specific* concept means that the practitioner prescribing the patient's pulmonary rehabilitation program must take into full consideration the patient's total lifestyle, both at home and at work. He then must design and implement a rehabilitation program that will be of the most direct, useful benefit to that patient. For example, if a patient's domestic chores included vacuuming, then the specific ROM and breathing pattern would need to be established for that activity. Another example, and one of universal application, would be teaching the patient the necessary energy-conserving motions applicable to personal hygiene needs. In this case, a different type of breathing pattern would need to be taught for combing one's hair as opposed to attending to toilet needs such as defecating.

The therapist who is teaching the patient the various activities must keep in mind that particular patient's needs and not mentally stereotype the patient or the activity to be taught. Sometimes the law of universality may not apply. (For example, teaching a patient how to brush his teeth in an energy-conserving fashion is a misdirected effort when the patient wears dentures and merely plops them into a bowl of effervescent solution each night!)

In summary, the concept of task-specific breathing training is a basic tenet of the principles, practice, and philosophy of pulmonary rehabilitation. All members of the pulmonary rehabilitation team must constantly keep the patient's lifestyle in mind and address that lifestyle when developing and implementing the patient's rehabilitative program. As each new modality is introduced, it never hurts to ask the patient, "Is this going to help you in your daily endeavors?" Also, if the talents of an occupational therapist are available, use them. The occupational therapist can be a valuable member of the pulmonary rehabilitation team.[1]

Psychosocial Considerations

In addition to physiologic impairment, the cognitive, affective, and psychomotor levels of ability of the patient must be evaluated and taken fully into account prior to initiating rehabilitative procedures of any kind. All three of these domains play an important role in the patient's ability to perform many of the physical tasks required in a rehabilitative program. Of equal importance are the patient's motivation, lifestyle, and general socioeconomic status (see Chapters 10 and 11). The practitioner is advised to keep these factors in mind when implementing the breathing training and exercise techniques to be discussed in the rest of this chapter. Those programs fortunate enough to have a total multidisciplinary approach may elect to use the psychological psychiatric and social service members of the team to help in the psychological and social evaluation of pulmonary rehabilitation candidates.

Breathing Training Techniques

Some of the basic types of breathing training maneuvers will now be presented. The whole regimen of breathing training techniques is virtually ad infinitum when one takes into account the previously introduced task-specific concept. Thus, the techniques to be introduced here are merely representative of the basic principles of breathing training and serve as the foundation from which the entrepreneurial practitioner can develop other training techniques that address each patient's particular needs.

Diaphragmatic Pursed-Lip Breathing

The overall physiologic benefit of D-PLB (Fig 6–1) is that it allows for a more effective breathing pattern and thus an improved ventilatory exchange on a breath-to-breath basis. Specific benefits include the following:

1. More effective oxygen intake (room air or supplemental oxygen) and CO_2 removal at the alveolar level.

2. Larger tidal volumes, which should decrease minute respiratory rate, increase minute ventilation, and reduce total wasted ventilation.

3. A reduction in unnecessary use of accessory respiratory muscle at rest and, to a degree, while exercising at submaximal loads.

4. A more rhythmic and cadence-type breathing that is not only physiologically, but also more psychologically satisfying.

5. A more aesthetically acceptable type of breathing that does not call as much public attention to the patient's affliction.

Initially, the patient will need to conscientiously practice D-PLB until it becomes a fixed, spontaneous method of breathing. Practice sessions of 5 to 10 minutes with close scrutiny by the therapist will help to reinforce the proper technique. Although the patient will be expected to incorporate D-PLB into his everyday life, repeat demonstrations during future outpatient clinic visits should be requested of the patient by the therapist. This intermittent supervision will help to confirm that the patient has mastered this breathing technique.

When possible, the therapist should observe the patient's breathing without bringing it to the patient's attention that he is being observed. This is really the only empiric method to ascertain that the patient is performing his D-PLB optimally. A common problem the patient will experience is that of developing a sense of inspiratory-to-expiratory timing. Senile or patients with chronic cerebral hypoxia will find it especially difficult to master

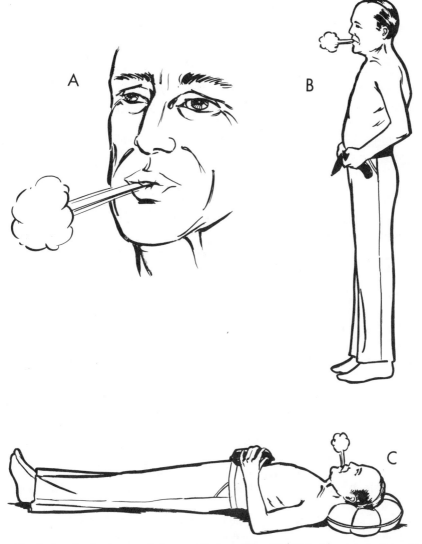

Fig 6–1.—A, diaphragmatic/pursed lip breathing (D-PLB). **B,** using belt to aid exhalation while doing D-PLB. **C,** recumbent position using sandbag to aid exhalation while doing D-PLB.

this technique to any degree of optimal performance. The therapist may need to use little tricks that will assist the patient in developing a sense of timing for physiologically proper inspiratory-expiratory (I:E) ratios. For example, a patient may find it useful to implement the standard technique of mentally counting to oneself ("one thousand-and-one, one thousand-and-two, one thousand-and-three . . .") during the inspiratory and expiratory phases of his breathing. The use of a timing pegboard is useful when initially teaching the patient I:E ratios to be used when bending over to tie his shoes or picking up dropped objects (Purdue Pegboard, LaFayette Instrument Co., LaFayette, Ind.).[1]

Does D-PLB really work? To what extent can its usefulness be measured? Scientific and empiric data is available. Scientific observations by Motley[2] in 1963 evaluated the efficacy of D-PLB for patients on positive pressure breathing therapy. Motley's experiment with 35 severe emphysema patients who were taught proper breathing techniques resulted in an average decrease in respiratory rate from 15.2 to 9.4 per minute. This resulted in an average tidal volume increase from 0.494 to 0.814 L per breath over a 3-minute sampling period. The resting arterial blood oxygen saturation was increased in all except two cases.

A study similar to Motley's was done by Mueller and coworkers[3] in 1970. Mueller's group reported that pursed lip breathing alone while at rest increased Pa_{O_2} and Sa_{O_2} while Pa_{CO_2} decreased. No improvement was seen during exercise. Interestingly enough, no effects on O_2 uptake, CO_2 production rates, physiologic deadspace, alveolar ventilation, alveolar-arterial gradient, P_{O_2} gradient or DL_{CO} were noted. Mueller used 12 patients in his study, 7 of which claimed relief while pursed lip breathing, and the other 5 denying any relief. Both groups did show improvements in arterial blood gas levels, however. Observations from Mueller's study included these comments:

1. Generally, D-PLB provides its greatest symptom benefit during and immediately after exertion; however, many note relief during rest as well.

2. D-PLB is a more effective form of breathing in the sense that during such a maneuver, less air has to be breathed to absorb a given amount of oxygen.

3. Symptom relief provided by D-PLB may be linked to the degree to which D-PLB increases tidal volume and decreases respiratory rate.

4. D-PLB improves arterial blood gases, but only at rest and in no relation to symptom relief.[3]

Are there any negative or untoward effects of D-PLB? Observations commented upon in Mueller's report stated that although there was a decrease in the V_{O_2} indicating a more effective form of breathing, the fact that the O_2 uptake remained unchanged meant that D-PLB provided no change in actual total body metabolic economy. Mueller also noted that the work of breathing per breath might actually be increased due to the active requirement of the patient to purse his lips, along with the influence of the expiratory resistence and increased tidal volumes ensuing. Ingram and Schilder in another study in 1967 concluded with the same observations and, like Mueller, believed that this supposed increased work of breathing is what may negate any direct benefits of increased O_2 uptake.[3]

Summarily, the positive effects of D-PLB are those noted by Motley and Mueller. The negative effects, in view of any "deleterious" possibilities, appear to be nonexistent. The only drawbacks to D-PLB may be the possibility of increased work of breathing associated with the body dexterity required to effectively perform the maneuver; however, the benefits would appear to more than offset any overt effort required of the patient.

Range of Motion

The basic principles of ROM activities for pulmonary rehabilitation patients are borrowed from physical medicine principles and adapted to the COLD patient's needs. However, instead of patient passivity as would be normally expected in conventional physical therapy, the pulmonary rehabilitation patient actively participates in the various abduction (movement of limbs away from the body) and adduction (movement of limbs toward the body) movements. Of course, the convalescing or semiambulant patient may require some assistance from the therapist, but the end goal is always to allow the patient to perform the movement independently.

When the patient has mastered the basics of the various ROMs (Fig 6–2), he can then transfer the training effects for use in the task-specific concept discussed earlier in this chapter. Some of the specific benefits of teaching the patient ROM are as follows:

1. When incorporated with D-PLB, allows the patient to pursue daily activities without undue dyspnea.

2. Teaches the patient to associate his daily activities with specific energy- and oxygen-conservative movements.

3. Allows for more efficient and effective movement with a greater net return of work unit gained per work unit performed.

4. Incorporates task-specific concept, which allows for a transfer of training effect.

5. Serves as a warm-up prior to exercise training.

6. Improves psychological outlook and morale due to patient's improved physical agility.

The ROMs illustrated in Figure 6–2 represent the basic abduction and adduction movements that will allow for a training transfer effect. These movements become more meaningful and useful to the patient when modified to fit his actual daily lifestyle. The patient's orthopedic limitations will need to be evaluated and limits set as necessary. Some patients will require close supervision and coaching due to lack of natural dexterity, senility, or decreased mentation due to chronic cerebral hypoxia. The patient should

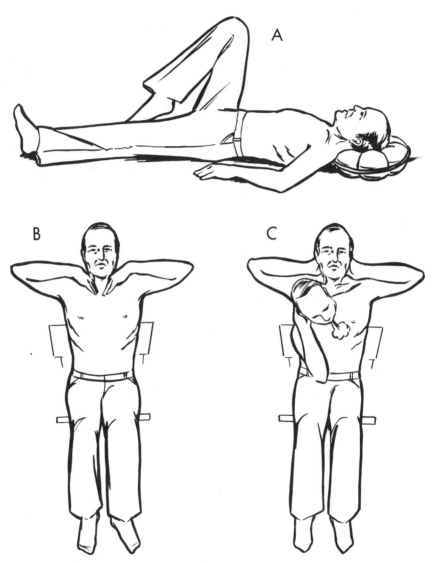

Fig 6–2.—ROM exercises. Cardinal principles: (1) incorporate D-PLB; (2) always exhale when "adducting," inhale when "abducting." **A,** kneebend: patient *exhales* while bringing knee toward chest and *inhales* when bringing knee to rest flat on table or bed. Alternate legs. **B,** modified arm raises: patient *inhales* while raising arms, *exhales* while lowering arms. **C,** elbow to knee: patient *exhales* while touching elbow to knee, *inhales* when returning to resting position. Alternate with other elbow and knee.

be encouraged to implement the ROM methods into his daily lifestyle as well as to implement new ROMs appropriate to his needs.

Principles of Exercise

Once the patient has mastered breathing training techniques to the best of his ability, he is then ready to begin a planned, supervised program of exercise as defined earlier. The patient, of course, should have had all the necessary cardiopulmonary stress testing, pulmonary function, and arterial blood gas studies completed prior to beginning any exercise program. It will be from these preexercise studies that an exercise prescription delineating physiologic limits can be determined (see Chapter 4).

The rehabilitative objectives of exercise are to (1) increase the capacity to do work, (2) increase maximum oxygen uptake, (3) increase endurance, i.e., total time spent exercising, and (4) increase blood flow to the muscle(s) being exercised. The net result of these objectives alone or together is to decrease the work of breathing for any given task.

Any exercise program prescribed should be able to meet all or most of the following criteria if the exercise is to be of a clinically evaluative as well as a direct physiologic benefit to the patient. These criteria are:

1. Able to be performed by most patients and simulates an activity normally undertaken in their daily lifestyle.

2. Can easily be duplicated at another time or locale for determining progress and documentation purposes.

3. Lends itself to measurement and recording of physiologic parameters when a test session is desired.

4. Is inexpensive to the patient when doing it on his own, and requires minimal preparation time and supervision.

5. Causes a true exercise training effect upon body, i.e., increased heart rate, increased ventilation, muscle toning, etc.

6. Allows for a transfer of training effect.

Walking, cycling (cycle ergometer, bicycle), stair climbing, and treadmill exercise fulfill the majority of these criteria. However, Belman and Wasserman,[4] citing Paez and associates' work[5] in 1967, commented that the beneficial effects of cycling may not transfer to walking. They believed it may be better to train the patient in a modality of exercise, i.e., walking, that is inherently useful in everyday activities. A review of the literature to date shows no exhaustive studies of walking or treadmill vs. cycling. Both treadmill and cycling allow for viable clinical testing for determining anaerobic thresholds and other respiratory parameters. European investigators, however, seem to favor the cycle ergometer for testing and bicycling as the preferred home exercise modality. This is probably a cultural preference, since the bicycle is a common mode of transportation and recreation in

Europe. Conversely, the fad for jogging, when translated into walking for patients, may be the preferred mode of exercise in the United States. Of course, some patients can obtain a dual benefit, especially in inclement weather, and use a stationary bicycle for in-home exercise.

Regarding the specific training and training transfer effects of the treadmill, Vyas and associates[6] cited the work of Paez and colleagues,[5] whose conclusion it was that improvement in performance on the treadmill might in fact be a spurious improvement due to curtailment of wasted movement and resulting in improved mechanical efficiency. Vyas' group also referred to others' works,[7, 8] and summarized that even the step test, like the treadmill, can involve variable amounts of unrecorded external work as well as other limitations.

Techniques of Exercise

When exercise training is earnestly initiated, the patient will need to have at his command the full range of breathing training techniques previously discussed. Not only do the two complement each other, but exercise training is difficult to initiate and sustain without previously mastering breathing training techniques.

Walking

The same basic principles of energy conservation and breathing coordination used in D-PLB and ROM are applied to walking. Walking is certainly not a new task to the patient; however, due to the gradual encroachment of his lung disease, the patient alters this activity to compensate for the physiologic changes that occur. The result of the patient's adaptive measures culminates in severely reduced mobility due to incorrect walking/breathing patterns and an asynchronous, energy-inefficient effort. It is not an uncommon sight to see the untrained COLD patient make a resting station of every stationary object as he pants his way to his first appointment. Ironically, the patient may psychologically believe that his breathing/walking pattern is perfect for him. A vicious cycle ensues. The end clinical picture is the patient, often stooping or bending over and supporting his breathing efforts by fixing his arm-shoulder-chest muscles (the "professorial" position), saying, "I feel fine and actually don't get short of breath . . . as long as I don't move from this position."

The specific benefits of teaching the patient proper walking techniques and encouraging him to walk daily are as follows:

1. Walking is coordinated with previously taught breathing patterns for maximal efficiency of ventilation.

2. Walking provides a mild-to-moderate stress exercise on the cardiopulmonary system.

TABLE 6–1.—TECHNIQUE FOR WALKING*

1. Patient begins by standing at a starting point where a premeasured distance has been marked off.
2. Take resting pulse.
3. The patient will already be doing D-PLB, which will ease him more naturally into the cadence and rhythm of walking in an energy-conservative fashion.
4. Starting off on the left foot, the patient walks at a stride and speed comfortable to him. He should mentally be counting out his I:E ratios to himself.
5. Patient walks a distance comfortable for him, stopping and resting as necessary, and starts walking again when he feels comfortable.
6. Take pulse at end of walk.
7. Fill out walking chart (Fig 6–4).

*Patient should already know how to perform D-PLB so it can be incorporated into walking.

3. Walking is vital to the success of the patient's daily life if his domestic or work situation demands mobility.

4. Walking provides a psychological sense of freedom and independence.

Table 6–1 outlines the technique for walking (Fig 6–3). Again, it is expected that the patient has already been taught breathing training techniques, especially D-PLB. Figure 6–4 is an example of a walking chart to be used by the patient for keeping a record of walking at home.

Twelve-Minute Walking Test

An excellent method of assessing pulmonary disability in regard to walking is by having the patient complete a 12-minute walking test. This test, originally described by Cooper[9] and modified for clinical use, measures the amount of ground covered in 12 minutes of continuous walking. McGavin and associates[10] used this test to assess disability in chronic bronchitis patients and believed the reproducibility of the test was valid and within defined and accepted limits. McGavin thought that the use of a standard time rather than a standard distance was more clinically representative of the patient's endurance and tolerance. Twelve minutes is also the appropriate length of time to test oxygen uptake for most patients.

Stair Climbing

Climbing stairs (Figs 6–5 and 6–6) not only provides exercise for the COLD patient, but also trains him for an activity he may be routinely called upon to do in his everyday life. Table 6–2 outlines the technique for stair climbing. The benefits of a stair climbing program for chronic bronchitis were described by McGavin and colleagues.[11] Their controlled trial showed that the stair climbing program in their specific study resulted in significant benefits in terms of general well-being and reduced breathlessness.

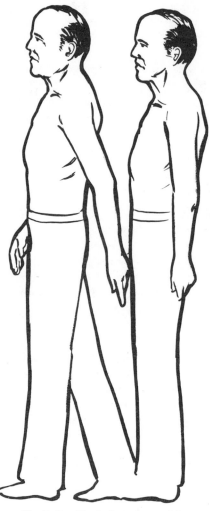

Fig 6–3.—Technique for walking.

Treadmill and Stationary Cycle

Clinically, the treadmill (Fig 6–7) and stationary cycle (Fig 6–8) ergo-meter serve a dual purpose. Initially, they serve as the testing devices for determining pulmonary thresholds. Both devices can then be implemented for further inpatient or outpatient use as exercise machines. Although all patients should be encouraged to walk, those preferring the stationary cy-cle should not be discouraged from purchasing one; however, they should

Date	Starting Time/ Finishing Time	Pulse: Before/After	Weather Conditions	How did you feel before walking?	How did you feel after walking?	Distance Walked

Fig 6–4.—Sample of a walking progress sheet.

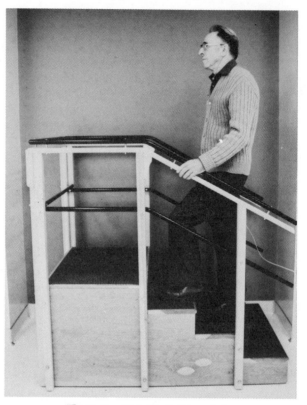

Fig 6–5.—Patient climbing stairs.

be encouraged to use the cycle as an augmentation to walking or as a substitute for walking during inclement weather. One benefit of using a stationary cycle is that if the patient's original pulmonary evaluation was on a cycle ergometer, then a reference point has already been established for lower and upper exercise limits. However, patients planning the preferred walking program (which will hopefully be the more likely choice) should

TABLE 6–2.—TECHNIQUE FOR STAIR CLIMBING*

1. Prior to starting up stairs, patient should be breathing in a rhythmic fashion using I : E ratios that will match climbing efforts.
2. Patient is instructed to exhale while stepping up and to inhale when foot comes to rest on each step.
3. Patient can stop and rest at any time while still on stairs. He should pause between each step he takes.

*D-PLB is incorporated into stair climbing.

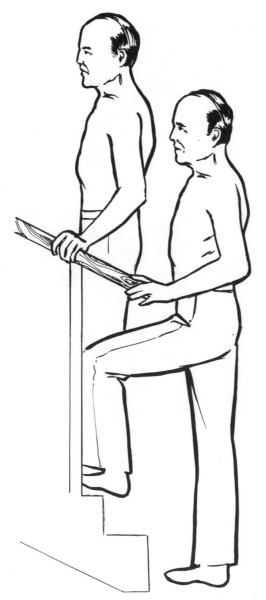

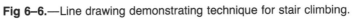

Fig 6–6.—Line drawing demonstrating technique for stair climbing.

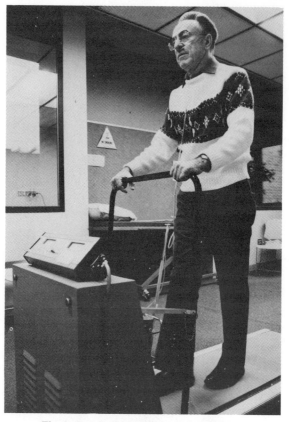

Fig 6–7.—Patient walking on treadmill.

still be able to gain benefit from the treadmill pulmonary evaluation and integrate it into their at-home walking program.

Writing the Exercise Prescription

After completion of the exercise evaluation as outlined in Chapter 3, an exercise prescription can be devised so that the patient can undertake an exercise regimen under more predictable terms than if he were to gauge his exercise limits by purely subjective feelings.

There are four components to an exercise prescription: (1) intensity, (2) duration, (3) frequency, and (4) mode.

1. *Intensity* of exercise is derived from the progressive work phase of the exercise evaluation. The maximum energy expenditure or $\dot{V}O_2$ and maximum heart rate (MHR) are the physiologic variables from which a target

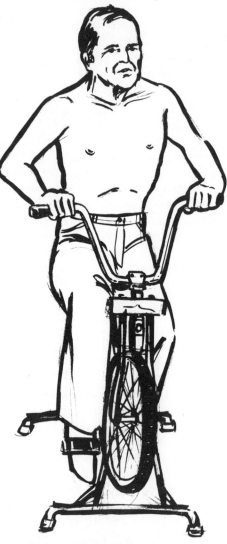

Fig 6–8.—Patient using exercycle.

heart rate is established. The goal of exercise is to start at a level of exercis̶ equal to 60% of the patient's maximum achieved $\dot{V}O_2$ and work up to 80 of the maximum $\dot{V}O_2$. A method of calculating this is as follows:

$$60\% \text{ of } \dot{V}O_2 \text{ max} = 70\% \text{ of predicted MHR}$$

Example

V_{O_2} max $= 1.2$ L/min
MHR predicted $= 180$
60% of 1.2 L/min $= 0.72$ L/min
70% of 180 MHR $= 126$, or the desired heart rate

The exercise load should be set to achieve a beginning heart rate of 126 beats per minute in the example. The load should be increased gradually until a "target heart rate" of 144 beats per minute ($\pm$ 5%) is achieved.

2. *Duration* of exercise should ideally reach a level of 20 to 30 minutes per session. Needless to say, the COLD patient cannot be expected to work for that amount of time at the onset of the program. He will need to proceed at his own pace and gradually increase his exercise time increments from 3 minutes to 5 minutes and so on.

3. *Frequency* is important and helps to determine the ultimate success of the patient's exercise benefits in terms of both objective and subjective fitness. The novice patient just starting in an exercise program will be doing exercise of less duration per session. Therefore, he should be encouraged to exercise more often. Two to three short periods of exercise consisting of 3 to 5 minute sessions each day would not be inappropriate.

4. *Mode* of exercise can consist of walking, cycling or stair climbing, which can be individually performed each session or combined. When feasible, it should be task specific, e.g., walk to the newspaper stand, store, etc.

Patients who are not on oxygen may require supplemental oxygen during exercise. Those already on oxygen may need to increase the flow by 1 to 2 L/min. For example, a patient with a resting Pa_{O_2} of 55 mm Hg and on continuous oxygen at 2 L/min may need to increase this to 3 to 4 L/min while exercising. Ear oximetry studies during exercise will assist in determining if a deleterious amount of oxygen desaturation is occurring.

Vyas and coworkers[12] noted particularly striking differences in the amount of exercise performed when patients on supplemental oxygen were compared with those breathing room air only. Vyas believed that other than an increase in P_{CO_2} levels of the supplemental oxygen group, this group was able to increase their work-load performance, and therefore the oxygen was a valuable adjunct to the patient's exercise program.

Are the exact mechanisms known by which supplemental oxygen allows the COLD patient to exercise to a greater degree than the room air-breathing patient? Belman and Wasserman,[4] reviewing others' studies,[13-16] indicated that while the oxygen helped, the exact mechanisms were not clearly known. One study from unpublished data attributed the increased exercise

tolerance to oxygen's effect on either the reduced ventilatory drive from the carotid bodies or to a decreased pulmonary artery pressure (see Chapter 7). Whatever the exact mechanism or combination of mechanisms may be, many investigators find oxygen to be of use in the patient's exercise program.

Summary

Do breathing training techniques and exercise programs do all that they are purported to do? Both empirically and scientifically, the answer appears to be yes. It must be kept in mind that the very subjective nature of the patient's dyspnea does not allow for any strict application of conventional scientific principles to quantify and qualify the results of his participation in a pulmonary rehabilitation program. Of course, laboratory datum such as the arterial blood gas analysis does give objective information and allows the practitioner to evaluate beyond the clinical symptoms overtly displayed by the patient.

What does breathing training and exercise do for the patient besides teaching proper breathing and providing cardiopulmonary exercise? The positive psychological benefits to be gained cannot be overemphasized. When the patient develops a better psychological outlook, then he is more likely to be spurred on to continue with the pulmonary rehabilitation program's physical demands. Agle and coworkers[17] observed that patients who were taught breathing training techniques believed they had more control over their destinies and were not as subject to the whims of dyspnea attacks. These patients also find out just how much dyspnea they can safely tolerate and thus are more likely to allow some lifting of self-imposed restraints.

The importance of teaching breathing training along with exercise cannot be overstressed. It is imperative that the clinician and patient alike understand the importance of these two facets and coordinate them into the total rehabilitative process. A study by Casciari and colleagues[18] showed that patients receiving breathing training instruction along with exercise showed an increase in exercise performance. Empiric observations and experiences by the author concur with and support the gross observations of Motley[2] and Mueller and associates[3] cited earlier. Although no conclusive studies have yet been completed, experiences to date at the author's institutions (Grandview Hospital and Southview Hospital and Family Health Center, Dayton, Ohio) would appear to bear out Casciari's, Motley's, and Mueller's observations.

One area of exercise the pulmonary rehabilitation practitioner will see develop into a more commonly used training modality is *inspiratory muscle training* (IMT).[19, 20] Basically, IMT is an exercise that builds up the inspiratory muscles. This is achieved by having the patient inspire through a mouthpiece capable of being adjusted to smaller increments via various size orifices that fit onto the mouthpiece. This mouthpiece/orifice restriction device is attached to two one-way valves. One valve permits inspiration through the restrictive orifice, thus achieving the desired IMT effect. The other valve is unrestricted and allows for natural exhalation to ambient pressures. One commercially produced IMT device is pictured in Figure 6–9. Its mechanism, located on the top of the device, is a series of gradually smaller holes. Orifice sizes may start at 0.47 cm in diameter and are gradually reduced to 0.24 cm or 0.18 cm in diameter by the end of a 6-week training period. The patients are instructed to use the device twice a day for 10- to 15-minute periods, graduating to 30 minutes as tolerated. The benefits of IMT are as follows:

1. Improvement of other types of exercise performance for an overall net effect greater than conventional pulmonary rehabilitative exercises.[20, 21]

2. Much larger increases in submaximal exercise endurance (as much as 64% in one study[20]).

Another area gaining recognition is *biofeedback*. Clinical psychologists have long used the concept of sound and light or other sensory awareness devices to aid in relaxation. The same concept can be applied to help teach COLD patients how to relax their ventilatory muscles for more effective,

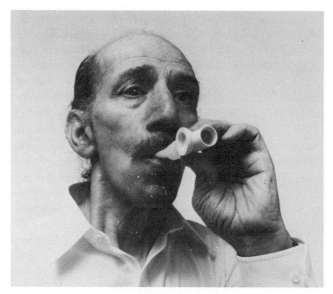

Fig 6–9.—Patient using IMT device. (Courtesy of Healthscan, Upper Montclair, N.J.)

efficient breathing. Biofeedback training can be a valuable adjunct therapy for the patient unable to monitor the effectiveness of his attempts at breathing control. It is especially helpful to those with the ability to perform diaphragmatic breathing but who still have a tendency to allow upper chest muscle breathing to override the more natural, ventilatory-superior effects of proper diaphragmatic excursion. Chapter 7 details the benefits of biofeedback.

Finally, it is important to remember that the science and art of pulmonary rehabilitation is in a constant state of change, which is as it should be if we are to reach an optimum level of care for this new discipline. Therefore, it would be impossible to list, illustrate, and describe every technique employable in the rehabilitative process of the COLD patient. Because of the new state of science and art of pulmonary rehabilitation, the techniques vary from institution to institution and are often reflective of an individual's or group's efforts and entrepreneurship.

References

1. Pomerantz P., Flannery E., Findling P.: Occupational therapy for chronic obstructive lung disease. *Am. J. Occup. Ther.* 29:407–411, 1975.
2. Motley H.L.: The effects of slow deep breathing on the blood gas exchange in emphysema. *Am. Rev. Respir. Dis.* 88:485–492, 1963.
3. Mueller R.E., Petty T.L., Filley G.F.: Ventilation and arterial blood gas exchange induced by pursed lips breathing. *J. Appl. Physiol.* 28:784–789, 1970.
4. Belman M.J., Wasserman K.: Exercise training and testing in patients with chronic obstructive pulmonary disease. *Basics Resp. Dis. Am. Lung Assoc.* 10:1–8, 1981.
5. Paez P.N., Phillipson E.A., Masangkay M., Sproul B.J.: The physiologic basis of training patients with emphysema. *Am. Rev. Respir. Dis.* 95:944–53, 1967.
6. Vyas M.N., Banister E.W., Morton J.W., Grzybowski S.: Response to exercise in patients with chronic airway obstruction: I. Effects of exercise training. *Am. Rev. Respir. Dis.* 103:390–399, 1971.
7. Cotes J.E.: *Lung Function.* Philadelphia, F.A. Davis, Co., 1966, p. 290.
8. Bates D.V., Christie, R.V.: *Respiratory Function in Disease.* Philadelphia, W.B. Saunders Co., 1964, p. 74.
9. Cooper K.H.: A means of assessing maximal oxygen intake. *JAMA* 203:135–138, 1968.
10. McGavin C.R., Gupta S.P., McHardy G.J.R.: Twelve-minute walking test for assessing disability in chronic bronchitis. *Br. Med. J.* 1:822–823, 1976.
11. McGavin C.R., Gupta S.P., Lloyd E.L., McHardy G.J.R.: Physical rehabilitation for the chronic bronchitic: Results of a controlled trial of exercises in the home. *Thorax* 32:307–311, 1977.
12. Vyas M.N., Banister E.W., Morton J.W., Grzybowski S.: Responses to exercise in patients with chronic airway obstruction: II. Effects of breathing 40 percent oxygen. *Am. Rev. Respir. Dis.* 103:401–412, 1971.
13. Oxygen in the home, editorial. *Br. Med. J.* 2:1909–1910, 1981.
14. Wasserman K.: Unpublished data.

15. Longo A.N., Moser K.M., Luchsinger P.C.: The role of oxygen therapy in the rehabilitation of patients with chronic obstructive lung disease. *Am. Rev. Respir. Dis.* 103:690–697, 1971.
16. Legget R.J.E., Flenley D.C.: Portable oxygen and exercise tolerance in patients with chronic hypoxic cor pulmonale. *Br. Med. J.* 2:84–86, 1979.
17. Agle D.P., Baum G.L., Chester E.H., et al.: Multidiscipline treatment of chronic pulmonary insufficiency: I. Psychological aspects of rehabilitation. *Psychosom. Med.* 35:41–49, 1973.
18. Casciari R.J., Fairshter R.D., Harrison A., et al.: Effects of breathing retraining in patients with chronic obstructive pulmonary disease. *Chest* 79:393–398, 1981.
19. Sonne L.J., Davis J.A.: Increased exercise performance in patients with severe COPD following inspiratory resistive training. *Chest* 81:436, 1982.
20. Pardy R.L., Rivington R.N., Despas P.J., Macklem P.T.: Inspiratory muscle training compared with physiotherapy in patients with chronic air flow limitation. *Am. Rev. Respir. Dis.* 123:421, 1981.
21. Belman M.J., Kendregan B.A.: Physical training fails to improve ventilatory muscle endurance in patients with chronic obstructive pulmonary disease. *Chest* 81:440, 1982.

7 / Biofeedback

JEROME E. HOLLIDAY, Ph.D.

THIS CHAPTER WILL PRESENT the underlying theory, techniques, and scientific evidence for the use of biofeedback in the patient with chronic obstructive lung disease (COLD). In addition, results will be given showing how other disciplines involved in pulmonary rehabilitation have used the patient's training in biofeedback to aid their efforts in pulmonary rehabilitation.

Biofeedback is basically a process by which information about some physiologic function that it is important for the patient to control is fed back to him through instrumentation. This means giving a patient immediate information about his or her own biologic condition, such as muscle tension, heart rate, and/or skin surface temperature. In some areas, biofeedback may be viewed with skepticism, particularly when it is considered as basic as exercise in pulmonary rehabilitation. Many experts in the field of pulmonary rehabilitation think in terms of exercise, but not relaxation. Some believe the COLD patient has become too sedentary, and muscle relaxation will only make him more lethargic. However, this is an oversimplified and superficial view of the COLD patient's situation. According to Jacobson,[1] a sedentary person can be a very tense person on the inside. In this chapter, evidence will be presented that reveals the COLD patient to be very tense and anxious, with many having a strong panic/fear reaction when they become short of breath. Putting a highly anxious patient through a rehabilitation exercise program without a muscle relaxation program could be detrimental to the patient.

There are other aspects to biofeedback besides muscle relaxation. As indicated above, biofeedback provides important information to the patient for bodily control. It is excellent for training mind-body interaction, because the patient comes to realize that fear of not getting a breath will cause muscle tightening and further shortness of breath. This chapter will demonstrate that breathing retraining, which is basic to any pulmonary rehabilitation program, can be improved with information provided by biofeedback to the patient.

85

Review of the Literature

The vast majority of scientific publications on the use of biofeedback for lung disease deals with asthmatics, and most of the articles and studies are on children. In general, biofeedback treatments involving asthmatics have sought to improve pulmonary function as an indication for reduction in airway resistance. Two approaches have been taken. The first is a direct one in which some measure of respiratory function is obtained, either peak flow rate (PEFR) or forced expiratory volume in 1 second (FEV_1), and the person given feedback about their function. The subject is then trained to change the measured parameters toward more normal levels. The second method is to effect an improvement in respiratory function by reducing muscle tension through frontalis electromyography (EMG) feedback and general relaxation. Davis and associates[2] were the first to report using a combination of frontalis EMG and Jacobson's relaxation to significantly increase PEFR for asthmatic children. There were three groups in their study: Group I received Jacobson's (1938) relaxation training with EMG feedback. Group II received Jacobson's relaxation training without feedback, and Group III, a control group, was provided with reading material and told to relax without any instruction. The subjects who received biofeedback and relaxation demonstrated greater improvement than those who received just relaxation.

In a slightly different design, Kotses and coworkers,[3] using only feedback, compared three different groups of asthmatic children for changes in PEFR. Group I received frontalis EMG feedback, Group II received pseudobiofeedback, and Group III was a no-treatment group. Only the group that received frontalis EMG feedback showed a significant increase in PEFR. In a subsequent study, Kotses and associates[4] compared EMG feedback from the frontalis muscle with EMG feedback from the arm (brachioradial muscle). Only feedback from the frontalis muscle showed a substantial change in PEFR. They concluded from this result that the ability of the skeletal musculature to influence PEFR resides primarily in facial muscles. Strangely, no comparison was made with the upper pectoral or intercostal muscles, which are the skeletal muscles directly involved in pulmonary function. This is probably due to the fact that the biofeedback-relaxation work on asthmatics performed by psychologists reflects thinking in terms of psychological relaxation rather than respiratory physiology.

The other approach reported in the literature is the use of feedback to give direct information on pulmonary function and how the asthmatics control respiratory function. Kahn and colleagues[5] induced bronchoconstriction in asthmatic children followed by training in bronchial dilation through feedback on FEV_1. The authors give no data on the actual changes in

FEV_1, but they did say that the majority of subjects controlled broncho-spasms within 10 minutes and reached their basal level. The authors report that the experimental group showed substantial reduction in medication frequency and hospital emergency room visits, the number of asthmatic attacks being reduced by half and the number of hospitalizations reduced from five to zero over a 10-month follow-up.

In a subsequent study, Kahn,[6] using a slightly modified procedure, sep-arated 80 asthmatic children into four groups, including an experimental and a control group, which were subdivided into reactors and nonreactors. Reactors were children who showed bronchoconstriction when it was sug-gested that they were being exposed to vapors to which they were allergic. Nonreactors showed no bronchoconstriction. The experimental groups of reactors and nonreactors both showed a 10% to 15% reduction in airway resistance. Over a 1-year period, both experimental groups showed a re-duction in numbers of attacks, duration of attacks, and the number of emergency room visits. It is interesting to note that the no-treatment re-active group showed similar symptom improvements.

There are two good reviews of the literature on the use of biofeedback on asthmatics, those of Olton and Noonberg[7] and Kotses and Glaus.[8] Even though the above results are very positive in regard to showing short-term (1 year or less) pulmonary symptom improvements in asthmatics with bio-feedback, Kotses and Glaus state that endorsement of biofeedback for asthma should be withheld until long-term improvement is obtained. Their attitude does not seem justifiable in light of the above results and is not the attitude taken by Olton and Noonberg, who state that asthma is a dis-order that may be successfully treated with biofeedback. In addition, many clinicians concerned with rehabilitation take the position that whatever helps the patient to function better should be used, despite the absence of objective studies of the efficacy of the techniques in question.

The results of Jacobson's[1] progressive relaxation to reduce airway resis-tance and asthmatic symptoms are not as impressive as the results of bio-feedback. The first experiment in this area was that of Alexander and col-leagues,[9] who found that 20 minutes of modified progressive relaxation resulted in a statistically significant 11% improvement in PEFR. However, in a more controlled study with improved measurements of pulmonary function, Alexander and associates[10] reported no significant improvement in pulmonary function or asthmatic symptoms with relaxation. Erskine and Schonell[11] reported no improvement in FEV_1 with progressive relaxation.

From the above results, it seems that biofeedback is producing other responses in addition to muscle relaxation. In a study using the locus of control scale on psychosomatic patients, Holliday and Munz[12] have sug-gested that what biofeedback was effecting beyond simple relaxation was giving the person a "sense of control" of his own body, or a belief that he could control his own body. Of course, this ability would be very important in pulmonary rehabilitation, particularly in the management of dyspnea.

Since the basic condition of asthma is the hypersensitivity of the airways to various external and internal stimuli, and because it is a reversible process, it is reasonable that control of airways is the major therapeutic consideration. The reversibility of the process is seen by the return of respiratory function to normal between asthma attacks. In emphysema, however, airway resistance results largely from structural damage and is not reversible. In contrast to the asthmatic, the emphysema patient's respiratory function does not return to normal between acute episodes in breathing. Thus, a different therapeutic intervention is needed for emphysema patients.

There are very few reports in the literature for the use of biofeedback or relaxation for the emphysema patient. In a case study, Broussard[13] reported using relaxation on an emphysema patient to determine the effect on heart rate, respiration rate, and blood pressure (BP). These parameters were recorded for 22 days prior to relaxation training and 14 days during relaxation protocol. The results showed a significant decrease in heart rate from 132 to 90 and respiration rate from 32 to 20. There was no significant change in BP.

Sitzman[14] used biofeedback to reduce respiration rate, for breathing retraining, and symptom control. Sitzman also reported using biofeedback for stress reduction in emphysema patients. Yanda[15] reported using EMG and Galvanic skin resistance biofeedback for tension reduction in COLD patients. Johnston and Lee[16] reported using EMG feedback from the external oblique muscle of the abdomen, and the lower rectus abdominis musculi for diaphragmatic breathing retraining. Their results showed that emphysema patients could learn diaphragmatic breathing more quickly and effectively through biofeedback than by conventional means.

From the above, the differences in the use of biofeedback for emphysema and asthmatics can be clearly seen. Biofeedback has been used for asthma to try to correct the basic pulmonary problem (airway resistance), while for emphysema it has been used as a therapeutic tool in rehabilitation and stress reduction.

There is some confusion in the terminology distinguishing emphysema (structural damage to lung airway resistance, not reversible), asthma (reversible airway resistance), and chronic bronchitis (mucous production, some reversibility of airway resistance). An individual can have any one or a combination of the above pulmonary disease processes, and the term COLD is used to cover all three. There are, however, some exceptions to this rule. Seldom do persons under 40 years of age develop significant emphysema. Since none of the subjects in the asthma studies were above 30 years of age, there was no component of emphysema in these studies. For the remainder of this chapter, the term COLD instead of emphysema, asthma, or chronic bronchitis will be used. However, the patients dealt with and the type of biofeedback interventions developed pertain primarily to those with an emphysema component of COLD.

The stress experienced by the COLD patient and its effect on their shortness of breath are not well understood or appreciated even by many in pulmonary rehabilitation. Broussard[13] states that the COLD person lives in a constant state of stress. They tend to be extremely nervous and tense, often not knowing if their next breath will come. Tension has the added effect of tightening the chest wall muscles, and thus making breathing more difficult. Dudley and coworkers[17] further emphasize the stress under which the COLD patient lives. They point out that the COLD patient lives in an emotional straightjacket. He cannot become angry, depressed, happy, or experience any other emotional change without risking the possibility of shortness of breath. Since anxiety and tension are strong factors in producing shortness of breath, relaxation will be a much more important factor in the management of emphysema than it is for asthma.

Anxiety and the COLD Patient

Dudley and associates[18] have stated that anxiety and depression are the most frequently encountered and perhaps the most disabling emotions accompanying COLD. This was also the main theme in the article cited above. Since shortness of breath can be greatly increased by nervousness and depression, special consideration should be given to the treatment of these conditions in pulmonary rehabilitation. Further support for this position is given by Hodgkin and colleagues,[19] who state that because of dyspnea and fear of suffocation, the COLD patient is likely to be tense and anxious. They further point out that in advanced stages the patient often assumes a body position to facilitate his breathing that may create further muscle tension.

At the pulmonary biofeedback laboratory at St. Louis University Hospital, we have found that many COLD patients report their shortness of breath is triggered by anxiety, while others state that they have never noticed any connection with shortness of breath. The lack of any observed connection by the subject may be due to denial, because many patients resent the implication that their physical distress has a connection with psychological problems. However, when it is made clear that psychological stress increases but does not directly cause shortness of breath, they often report later that they were surprised to learn from their own observations that shortness of breath can be triggered by stress.

Although it has been determined from clinical observations that COLD patients are very anxious, there has been little data or research studies to support this position. The biofeedback studies cited above were not research studies, but were mostly brief notes about using biofeedback on COLD patients. In a study by Holliday and associates,[20] it was shown that COLD patients are more anxious than chronically anxious patients. The basic reason for the anxiety in both the chronically anxious and the COLD patient is the fear of the consequence of expressing their own emotions. For the chronically anxious, it is the fear of social punishment, and for the COLD patient it is the fear of shortness of breath. However, the chronically anxious person can discharge his emotional impulses in the catharsis of rage or sex, while these avenues are not usually open to the COLD patient without becoming short of breath. It was thus hypothesized that the COLD patient would show greater psychological tension than the chronically anxious.

Research Study on COLD Anxiety

In this research study by Holliday and colleagues,[20] 14 COLD patients whose lung diseases were predominantly emphysema were compared with 10 chronically anxious patients. The chronically anxious patients had psychological symptoms of phobias, compulsions, excessive sweating, minor aches and pains, headaches, and muscular twitching of a year or more in duration. The degree of emphysema in the COLD patients was determined by pulmonary function studies, physical examination, and exercise testing at St. Louis University Hospital. All of the COLD patients had a FEV_1/FVC (forced vital capacity) ratio of less than 70% and a FEV_1 of less than 60% of predicted. In the COLD group, there were eight females and seven males, with an average age of 58. In the chronically anxious group, there were six females and four males, with an average age of 51. (It is important that the groups be closely balanced in regard to age and sex, because EMG is affected by both age and sex.) The 15 COLD patients were persons admitted between January and October 1982. The chronically anxious patients were those referred for biofeedback during this period.

In order to accurately compare the relative amount of anxiety and depression between the two groups, they were given the Beck depression scale, the Profile of Mood States (POMS), and a biofeedback diagnostic. The diagnostic compared the groups on baseline, biofeedback relaxation, and stress. There were five phases to the biofeedback diagnostic, lasting 5 minutes per phase. During the diagnostic, the physiologic parameters of frontalis EMG, upper pectoral EMG, diaphragmatic EMG (from intercostal muscles over diaphragm, COLD only), right and left finger temperature, right and left skin conductivity (SC), BP, and heart rate were measured. The placement of the electrodes on the patient is shown in Figures

7–1 and 7–2. The feedback was only from the frontalis muscle. Because the right and left hand may have different temperatures and SC, both hands were measured, and the highest value obtained was the measure used in the groups. The frontalis and upper pectoral muscles were measured on two Autogen 1700s,* and the diaphragmatic EMG was measured on an Autogen HT-1.* The SC was measured on two Autogen 3400s* and skin temperature on two Autogen HT-2s.* Data was accumulated on Expanded Technologies' Rockwell AIM-65, MDRS500.† This biofeedback equipment is shown in Figure 7–3. It is important to identify the instruments used, because measurements vary from one manufacturer to another, especially EMG measurements.

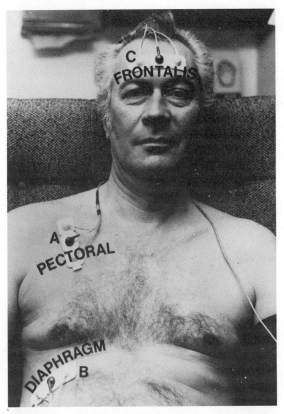

Fig 7–1.—Placement of EMG surface electrodes on patient to obtain EMG feedback from upper pectoral (A), diaphragm (B), and frontalis (C).

---

*Autogenic Systems, Inc., Berkeley, Calif.
†Expanded Technologies, Inc., Shreveport, La.

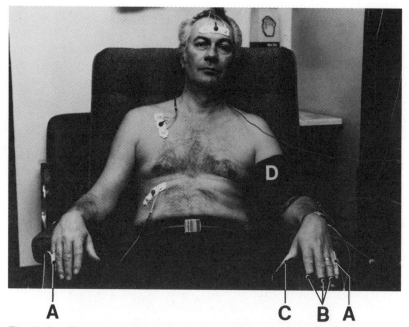

Fig 7–2.—Finger thermistor probes *(A)*. Skin conductivity electrodes *(B)*. Heart rate monitor *(C)*. Blood pressure cuff *(D)*.

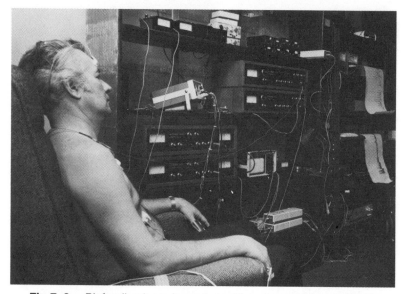

Fig 7–3.—Biofeedback equipment used in pulmonary biofeedback.

The first phase of the diagnostic was a baseline (B) phase in which the patients discussed hobbies or ways of relaxing. The second phase was a biofeedback-orientation phase (2-BF) in which patients received visual feedback about their frontalis muscle tension from the microvoltmeter in the Autogenic 1700. In this phase they experimented with various strategies to cause the meter to read lower (frontalis relaxed) or higher (increasing tension). They learned that anxious thoughts cause their forehead muscles to tighten up, and pleasant thoughts usually cause relaxation of these muscles. In the third phase, the patients received auditory EMG feedback (3-BF) in the form of clicks and were told to reduce the click frequency using the strategies learned in phase 2. Phase 4 was a stress phase (4-S) in which the patients self-disclosed on stressful topics. The fifth phase used auditory EMG feedback (5-BF) and was a repeat of phase 3. Phases 3 and 5 were used to compare the COLD patients' abilities to relax after stress with those of the chronically anxious patients. After each phase of the diagnostic, the patients were asked to rate their subjective feelings during the diagnostic phase on a scale of 0 to 10 (Table 7–1). The gradation of the scale is as follows: 0 to 4, states of decreasing relaxation; 5, normal feelings; and 6 to 10, states of increasing tension.

Because multivariant measures are being compared between the groups, the α value considered to indicate significance will have to be divided by the number of separate measurements (c) to determine the α level for significance when using dependent t measures. Because there are five separate measurements in the diagnostic profile, an α of .01 will have to be obtained to indicate significance at the .05 level ($\alpha c = .01 \times 5$), which is a Bonferroni inequality.[21]

Table 7–2 is a comparison of the EMG values for the frontalis and upper pectoral muscles as a function of the biofeedback diagnostic for COLD and chronically anxious patients. Using the independent multiple measure t test, there was a significantly ($P < .05$) greater frontalis and upper pectoral EMG at the base and stress phases of the diagnostic.

TABLE 7–1.—SUBJECTIVE FEELING SCALE

↑ Tension	10. Panic
	9. Very agitated
	8. Anxious, irritated
	7. Tense, upset
	6. Slightly tense, little uneasy
	5. Normal feelings
	4. Slightly relaxed, pleasant
	3. Muscles relaxed
Relaxation ↓	2. Passive, muscles heavy
	1. Drifting, floating
	0. Asleep

TABLE 7–2.—MEAN INTEGRATED EMG VALUES IN μV FOR
FRONTALIS AND UPPER PECTORAL MUSCLES DURING THE
DIAGNOSTIC USING FRONTALIS EMG FEEDBACK

	BIOFEEDBACK DIAGNOSTIC PHASES				
	1-B	2-BF	3-BF	4-S	5-BF
COLD					
Frontalis	7.30	4.01	2.36	6.58	2.59
Upper Pectoral	3.89	3.24	2.54	4.51	2.45
CHRONIC ANXIETY					
Frontalis	4.26	3.13	1.69	3.99	1.60
Upper Pectoral	2.04	1.88	1.55	2.15	1.41

This result shows that COLD patients have significantly ($P<$ .05) higher frontalis and pectoral muscle tension than the chronically anxious patients. Higher pectoral muscle tension might be expected for the COLD patient, because they are always struggling for breath. However, the higher frontalis muscle tension for the COLD patients suggests higher anxiety states, in view of the fact that the frontalis muscle is not involved in the respiratory disease.

Table 7–3 plots the BP for COLD patients as compared with those of the chronically anxious patients. There was no significant difference for baseline, but there was a significant difference ($P<$ .05) for subsequent sessions in the diagnostic profile. The BP data in Table 7–3 indicates that chronically anxious patients are able to reduce their BP with frontalis EMG feedback, but COLD patients are not. A similar situation is seen for the finger temperature of the two groups, shown in Figure 7–4. There is no significant difference for baseline, but there was a significant difference ($P<$ .05) for the first two frontalis EMG sessions and the stress sessions. Significance was not reached in the final session. These results indicate that as far as the autonomic nervous system is concerned, the COLD patients have a more difficult time relaxing than the chronically anxious patients. The heart rates of the two groups are plotted in Table 7–4, but there was no significant difference in the heart rates for any of the diagnostic phases

TABLE 7–3.—COMPARISON OF BP BETWEEN COLD
AND CHRONICALLY ANXIOUS PATIENTS*

	BIOFEEDBACK DIAGNOSTIC PHASES				
	1-B	2-BF	3-BF	4-S	5-BF
COLD	133/79	132/81	129/80	150/88	144/88
Chronically anxious	120/80	116/77	113/80	115/79	115/80

*Blood pressure taken at end of each diagnostic phase using frontalis EMG feedback.

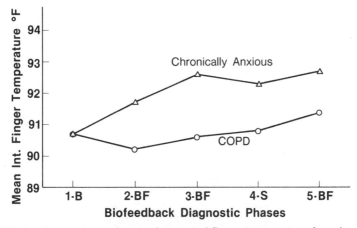

Fig 7-4.—Comparison of mean integrated finger temperature from hand with highest finger temperature as a function of biofeedback diagnostic phases between COLD patients and chronically anxious patients. (From Holliday J.E., Ruppel G., McDaniels S.: Comparison of biofeedback emphysema patients and chronically anxious patients, in Proceedings of the Fourteenth Annual Meeting of the Biofeedback Society of America. Denver, 1983, pp. 107–110. Used by permission.)

because of the large SD. However, the trend in heart rate is similar to finger temperature in that the heart rate moves toward the parasympathetic for the chronically anxious with biofeedback, but not for the COLD patient. COLD patients were, however, able to significantly reduce their frontalis and pectoral EMG with frontalis EMG feedback. This is shown in Figures 7–5 and 7–6, where frontalis and pectoral EMG are plotted as a function of the diagnostic phases. The fact that the COLD patients are able to reduce chest muscle tension can be an important factor in controlling dyspnea, as will be shown later. Using the αc criterion and dependent measures t test, there was a significant ($\alpha c = .05$) reduction for the COLD and chronically anxious patients in going from baseline and stress phases to

TABLE 7–4.—MEAN INTEGRATED HEART RATE FOR
BIOFEEDBACK DIAGNOSTIC PHASES COMPARING COLD
PATIENTS AND CHRONICALLY ANXIOUS PATIENTS
USING FRONTALIS EMG FEEDBACK

	BIOFEEDBACK DIAGNOSTIC PHASES				
	1-B	2-BF	3-BF	4-S	5-BF
COLD	87	88	86	90	87
Chronically anxious	81	76	76	78	75

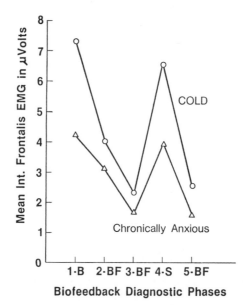

Fig 7–5.—The mean integrated frontalis EMG as a function of biofeedback diagnostic phase for frontalis EMG feedback. There was a significant difference ($P < .05$) in EMG values between COLD patients and chronically anxious patients. (From Holliday J.E., Ruppel G., McDaniels S.: Comparison of biofeedback emphysema patients and chronically anxious patients, in Proceedings of the Fourteenth Annual Meeting of the Biofeedback Society of America. Denver, 1983, pp. 107–110. Used by permission.)

the biofeedback phases for both frontalis and upper pectoral muscles EMG. The diaphragmatic EMGs for the COLD patient as a function of diagnostic phase is shown in Table 7–5. There was no significant difference between baseline and stress and the biofeedback phases as there was for frontalis and pectoral EMG.

The above results reported by Holliday and colleagues[20] show that COLD patients were highly anxious, with greather muscle tension than the chronically anxious person. The fact that muscle relaxation did not result

TABLE 7–5.—MEAN INTEGRATED
EMG VALUES IN µV FROM
INTERCOSTAL MUSCLES OVER
DIAPHRAGM FOR COLD PATIENTS

BIOFEEDBACK DIAGNOSTIC PHASES				
1-B	2-BF	3-BF	4-S	5-FB
3.18	2.89	2.78	3.21	2.64

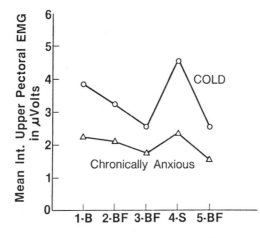

Biofeedback Diagnostic Phases

Fig 7–6.—The mean integrated upper pectoral EMG as a function of biofeedback diagnostic phases for frontalis EMG feedback. There was a significant ($P <$ .05) difference between the COLD and chronically anxious patients. (From Holliday J.E., Ruppel G., McDaniels S.: Comparison of biofeedback emphysema patients and chronically anxious patients, in Proceedings of the Fourteenth Annual Meeting of the Biofeedback Society of America. Denver, 1983, pp. 107–110. Used by permission.)

in shifting the autonomic nervous system from sympathetic dominance, as it did to some extent for the chronically anxious, shows the rigidity of the COLD patient. This result supports the "straightjacket"[17] concept of the COLD patient.

As indicated above[18] both anxiety and depression need to be dealt with in the COLD patient. The mean Beck depression scores for the COLD and chronically anxious patient was 10.9 and 10.2 respectively. A score of between 10 and 15 indicates a mild depression. If it is considered that at least three of the questions on the Beck test relate to physical symptoms likely to be experienced by the COLD patient, part of the mean depression score of the COLD patient could be accounted for as straightforward symptom reporting. There were three subscales of interest on the POMS, and the mean score of these three subscales is plotted in Figure 7–7. The tension scale has a higher T score than either anger or depression, and it is approximately one SD above that of depression, indicating that the COLD patient is more tense than he is depressed.

Some idea of the relative amount of depression or anxiety can also be obtained from the biofeedback diagnostic. If the physiologic parameters for the biofeedback phase after stress (phase 5) indicate less of a relaxed state

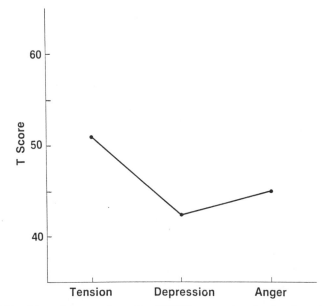

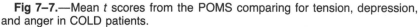

Fig 7-7.—Mean *t* scores from the POMS comparing for tension, depression, and anger in COLD patients.

than for the biofeedback phase before stress (phase 3), an anxiety state is indicated. This suggests the patient has difficulty in getting rid of troublesome thoughts and other tensions. If the person is more relaxed during phase 5 than in the biofeedback session before stress (phase 3), it is an indication of possible depression. Thus, the results indicate that getting feelings out helps to reduce depression and aids relaxation. For the 15 COLD patients, only 3 indicated a greater relaxed state after stress, and 2 of these showed extremely high muscle tension suggesting a great deal of tension along with possible depression.

The results indicate that anxiety is of much greater importance than depression in COLD. This gives strong justification for giving every COLD patient in a pulmonary rehabilitation program a biofeedback diagnostic to quantify the amount of the anxiety and tension.

Biofeedback for Controlling Dyspnea and Anxiety

In the previous section, scientific evidence[20] was presented that supported the clinical observations that COLD patients are highly anxious and tense and that pulmonary rehabilitation programs should include a biofeedback relaxation program. This should not be a program where only the most anxious COLD patients get referred to biofeedback, but the degree of anxiety shown by Holliday and colleagues[20] indicates that most pulmonary patients can expect to improve their ability to handle anxiety and dyspnea from biofeedback. The reduction of anxiety and dyspnea for the COLD patient results from learning control over his body. Gaarder[22] has stated that a variable cannot be controlled unless information is available about the variable. In the COLD patient's case, the variable is the body and the information is provided by biofeedback. The following information is given to the COLD patient by biofeedback in order to reduce his tension and anxiety and to control his dyspnea:

1. Information on how to relax in general and how to relax specific areas of the body.

2. Information on how to relax during activity.

3. Information on the effect of anxious thoughts on the body.

4. Information on the tension in the body (where it is and when it occurs).

5. Information from the diaphragm, chest, and accessory muscles for breathing retraining.

Thus, biofeedback provides more than just relaxation for the COLD patient; it provides extensive information enabling the COLD patient to control his own body. Many of the early papers on biofeedback, such as those of Green and coworkers[23] and Basmajian and colleagues,[24] showed that biofeedback could teach relaxation much faster and in greater depth than was possible by conventional techniques. This was because the person had information as to which techniques were effective in relaxation and which were not, as well as knowledge regarding the depth of his relaxed state. It might be argued that a person should know when he is relaxed or when he is not. However, many persons, such as those with COLD, have become used to such a high state of tension that they have no idea what a relaxed state feels like.

The key to relaxation and bodily control is to learn what William James[25] called the "passive will," i.e., the willingness to let things happen. This is sometimes called attention without effort. Passive volition is not part of our cultural training. We are trained to be assertive, to succeed, and to resist those forces that prevent us from doing what we wish. This resistance happens in shortness of breath when the person with COLD resists the shortness of breath and gets more short of breath. At the pulmonary biofeedback laboratory, we have found that the best way to teach passive volition is with biofeedback. In phase 2 of the biofeedback diagnostic, the COLD person is told to try hard to relax. In general, he will see a meter indicating increased tension. He is then told he cannot try to relax, but has to let go and not try. It would be very difficult to convey the passive will concept without biofeedback. This concept is then associated with shortness of breath, where it is pointed out that similarly if one tries too hard to get one's breath, the tension will increase and the shortness of breath will get worse.

At the end of each phase of the diagnostic, the patient is asked to rate his feelings on a scale of 0 to 10 (Table 7–1). Many times, his self-report of feelings is either more tense or more relaxed than indicated by the physiologic measurements. The COLD patient is then trained in greater body awareness. The lack of mind-body awareness is seen particularly after the stress session. When asked how he feels after self-disclosing on a stressful topic, he will report 6 or 7 on the subjective feeling scale. However, when asked how his body feels, he will say at first "okay," then on closer examination will relate that there is some tension. Further training in body awareness and control is provided with home progressive relaxation tapes. The patient is asked to practice these tapes once a day and to keep a daily log of his relaxation and how often he uses biofeedback to control dyspnea. He first learns to feel the tension he heard and saw with the EMG feedback instrument. This is important, because he cannot carry the instrument around with him to tell him when he is tense. The progressive relaxation tape teaches tensing and relaxing specific muscles. He learns the feel of these two states. From the feedback signal, he learns that very small changes in muscle tension produce changes in the feedback signal. The awareness gained from the feedback signal helps him to become more aware of tension before it might trigger shortness of breath. Table 7–1 lists the mean EMG values of the upper pectoral muscle. Values that are well above the mean indicate possible strong panic/fear reaction. However, if the COLD patient learns to become aware of this tension before it becomes too great, the panic/fear reaction can be avoided. To aid in the above process, the patient is also given a tape on Jacobson's differential relaxation. With this tape, he learns to relax the chest while using other muscles in walking or driving a car. As indicated earlier, COLD patients tend to walk tense with their shoulders high, which puts tension on the chest and makes breathing more difficult. Since a tense muscle will require more oxygen than a relaxed one, it is important that the COLD patient is tensing only those muscles required for the activity he is engaged in.

After the biofeedback diagnostic in which the COLD patient has learned the principle of muscle control and relaxation, as well as awareness of the contrast between tension and relaxation, the next step is upper pectoral or chest relaxation. One of the reasons for using frontalis EMG feedback in the biofeedback diagnostic rather than upper pectoral EMG feedback is that when the COLD patient first tries to relax his chest, he usually becomes tense. This increased tension is observed in several different physiologic parameters. When the patient is first given EMG feedback from the chest, there is sometimes an increase in chest tension over that for frontalis EMG feedback. There may also be an increase in SC and reduction in finger temperature during upper pectoral EMG feedback compared with frontalis EMG feedback.

In order to determine if COLD patients could effectively reduce upper pectoral muscle tension, the 15 patients in the research study were given four upper pectoral EMG feedback sessions (12 completed all four biofeedback sessions). Chest relaxation is not only important for improved breathing, but also basic to learning diaphragmatic breathing. Figure 7–8 shows the results of the study by Holliday and colleagues.[20] There was a significant ($P<.05$) decrease in upper pectoral EMG for the fourth biofeedback session relative to the first upper pectoral EMG feedback session, indicating that EMG biofeedback is an important method of relaxing and reducing tension for the COLD patient. As a result of this study, each patient in our pulmonary rehabilitation program at St. Louis University Hospital receives four sessions of upper pectoral EMG biofeedback beyond the diagnostic. However, for extremely anxious COLD patients, 12 sessions of biofeedback are recommended.

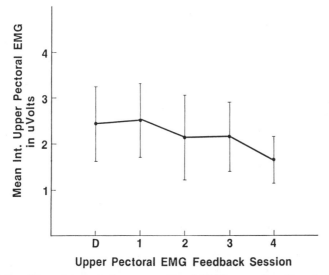

Fig 7–8.—Mean integrated upper pectoral EMG as a function of diagnostic *(D)* and upper pectoral EMG feedback sessions. There was a significant ($P <$ .05) drop in upper pectoral EMG for the fourth biofeedback session. (From Holliday J.E., Ruppel G., McDaniels S.: Comparison of biofeedback emphysema patients and chronically anxious patients, in Proceedings of the Fourteenth Annual Meeting of the Biofeedback Society of America. Denver, 1983, pp. 107–110. Used by permission.)

All 12 of the COLD patients reported that with the above biofeedback training they had less shortness of breath and were better able to abort a number of incidents of shortness of breath than before training. One patient reported being able to clean the living room without stopping, while before training she had to stop at least twice. Another patient reported a reduction in the use of inhaled bronchodilators (this patient had been using the bronchodilator seven times a day instead of the prescribed four). In addition, many COLD patients using biofeedback training are able to modify changes in heart rate or BP while performing conditioning exercises on cycle or ergometers. This is an important achievement for the patient, because it allows exercise training to continue in instances where it might have otherwise been terminated.

Breathing Retraining with Biofeedback

Hodgkin and colleagues[19] and Petty and coworkers[26] point out that the object of breathing retraining is to retrain the diaphragm so that (1) it becomes the main respiratory muscle, rather than accessory muscles, in order to decrease the energy required for breathing, (2) the respiratory rate is decreased; (3) the breathing pattern is coordinated so that the inhalation cycle will not commence before the exhalation cycle is completed; and (4) the 1:4 ratio is established between inhalation and exhalation and relaxed during exhalation. These objectives of breathing retraining were discussed by O'Ryan in Chapter 6, who mentioned that previously there was no effective method of training the patient in coordinated breathing so that the exhalation time was approximately four times that of inhalation.

According to Hodgkin and associates,[19] when the lung is functioning properly, 70% of the work of breathing is performed by the diaphragm and 30% is performed by the accessory muscles. In emphysema, however, the lung loses its elastic recoiling properties and becomes distended, which weakens and depresses the diaphragm. The flattened and weakened diaphragm is unable to ascend against the extended lung. In order to maintain pulmonary ventilation, the accessory muscles now account for about 70% of the breathing and the diaphragm only about 30%. The basic aim of breathing retraining according to Hodgkin and coworkers[19] is to restore the 70% diaphragm/30% upper pectoral and other accessory muscles ratio.

The first step in breathing retraining is to strengthen the diaphragm by expanding the abdomen and ribs on each inhalation. The usual method for the patient to sense movement of the diaphragm is by placing his hand on the diaphragm. However, by giving him EMG feedback from the area of the diaphragm (Fig 7–1), he can sense the movement of his diaphragm from the auditory feedback signal. The feedback information is used in reverse of that for relaxation. Instead of trying to keep the auditory signal off, he is trying to have it come on during inhalation. The amount that the patient moves the diaphragm can be controlled by the threshold value of the biofeedback instrument. The threshold is the value at which the feedback signal is first heard. As the threshold is increased, the COLD patient has to expand the abdomen further to turn on the feedback signal. It is important, however, that in a given biofeedback session he turns on the biofeedback signal to the same intensity so that a regular rhythm is developed. It is also important that the auditory feedback signal be turned off on each exhalation. The turning off of the signal tells the COLD person that he is relaxing his diaphragm on each exhalation. Petty and coworkers[26] emphasize that respiration must be done in a relaxed state and not be forced. By noting the time intervals between each inhalation, the patient can learn to reduce his respiration rate. A 1:4 ratio between exhalation and inhalation can be obtained by using diaphragmatic EMG feedback and the bitone derivative feedback on the Autogen 1700 Myograph Analyzer. When the patient is inhaling, a high-pitched tone will be heard (EMG level increasing), and a low-pitched tone will be heard on exhalation (EMG level decreasing). The COLD patient is instructed that he should hear the low-pitched tone approximately four times longer than the high-pitched tone. The feedback should be given with the threshold set at zero. Bitone derivative feedback cannot be used to strengthen the diaphragm, because it does not give information on EMG level, only on change in EMG muscle activity. The bitone derivative feedback aids in establishing coordinated breathing patterns.

The next step in breathing retraining is to reduce the muscle activity of the upper pectoral and accessory muscles. The basic principle of relaxing the upper pectoral muscle has been given in the previous section. As indicated earlier, there are two components to the upper pectoral EMG. These two components (A and B) are illustrated in Figure 7–9. In breathing retraining, it is the breathing component (A) of the EMG that one wants to reduce. When the COLD patient learns control of the chest EMG, he is next given EMG feedback simultaneously from both the upper pectoral and diaphragm. The training goal is to have the COLD patient keep the upper pectoral feedback signal off and the diaphragm signal on during inhalation.

In addition to providing information to the pulmonary rehabilitation patient for learning diaphragmatic breathing, data is obtained for quantitatively determining the patient's progress, which is not possible with present methods. By taking the following ratio, it is possible to determine if the patient is improving in diaphragmatic breathing (this ratio should increase with each biofeedback session):

Diaphragmatic EMG in μV/Pectoral EMG in μV

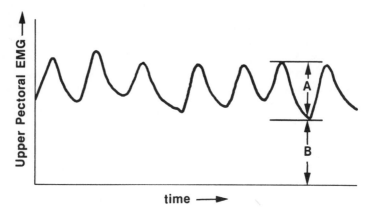

Fig 7–9.—Chest recording of rectified upper pectoral EMG showing the two components of the EMG: the expansion and contraction of the chest during breathing *(A)*, and that part of the upper pectoral EMG due to tension in the chest *(B)*.

Resistance Breathing

If the diaphragm has been weakened to a large extent by the distended lung, the above diaphragmatic exercise may not be sufficient to restore the diaphragm as the main respiratory muscle. Tests should be given to pulmonary patients to determine the fatigue point of the diaphragm. Muscle fatigue can be determined from the EMG of the muscle. The EMG of a muscle is a complex pattern of electrical impulses[27] that covers a frequency about 20 to 500 cycles. In EMG feedback, the electrical impulses are first amplified, then rectified and integrated, and then rendered in the form of auditory patterns and visual displays. However, in muscle-fatigue testing, the unrectified raw EMG is required. In advanced EMG feedback instruments, an output for the unrectified EMG is usually provided.

Kaiser and Petersen[28] have shown that muscle fatigue can be detected by demonstrating a shift in the frequency spectrum of the EMG of the fatigued muscle to lower frequencies. The amplitude of the low-frequency components of the EMG increases as the fatigue develops, while that of the high-frequency component decreases. Gross and coworkers[29] reported measuring diaphragmatic fatigue by placing surface electrodes on the sixth and seventh intercostal spaces. They have shown that fatigue of the diaphragm muscle can be obtained by measuring the fatigue of the intercostal muscles.

The unrectified EMG signal is passed through two ban pass filters with ranges of 20 to 45 Hz for the low-frequency component (L) and 150 to 300 Hz for the high-frequency component (H).

The H and L EMG signals are then recorded on a multichannel re-
corder. The amplitude of each H and L EMG for each breath is obtained
from the recording, and an H/L ratio is obtained for each breath. The H/L
ratio is then normalized against the initial H/L ratio, and a plot is obtained
of the H/L percentages of the initial values as a function of the number of
breaths. If the diaphragm is fatiguing, then the H/L ratio will decrease with
the number of breaths. If it is not fatiguing, the H/L ratio will remain
relatively constant.[28]

To test for diaphragmatic fatigue, the COLD patient breathes through a
restricted opening connected to the inspiratory inlet of a one-way breathing
valve. The EMG recordings are made for no resistance (baseline) and two
progressively higher resistances for 5 minutes each. The initial resistance
is chosen to induce approximately 30% maximal inspiratory mouth pressure. Inspiratory resistance is varied by changing the diameter of the inspiratory inlet opening. At the pulmonary biofeedback laboratory, it has
been found that for COLD patients the typical initial inlet sizes to elicit
fatigue are between 3 and 4 mm. A plot of the H/L percentage of the initial
value as a function of number of breaths for a COLD patient is shown in
Figure 7–10 for no resistance (normal breathing), a 3-mm inlet and a 2-mm
inlet opening. There is considerable variability in the H/L ratio between
breaths. It may be seen, however, that there was no downward trend in
the H/L ratio for normal breathing or for a 3-mm inlet opening. In fact, at
the end of the 5-minute session, there was an upward trend in the H/L
ratio for normal breathing. However, for the 2-mm inlet opening, there
was a definite downward trend indicating diaphragmatic fatigue. After 4
weeks of practice with inspiratory resistance breathing twice a day for 15
minutes using a 2 mm-inlet opening, the H/L ratio was measured again for
the same resistance. The results are shown in Figure 7–11, and no downward trend is observed in the H/L ratio, indicating no diaphragmatic fatigue after 4 weeks of resistance breathing practice.

The integrated upper pectoral EMG for the four resistance breathing
tests is listed in Table 7–6. It will be seen from the table that when the 2-
mm resistance produced fatigue, the upper pectoral accessory muscles
were the main respiratory muscles shown by the high EMG. However,
when the diaphragm was not fatiguing for a 2-mm inlet opening on resistance, the upper pectoral EMG dropped 68%, indicating the diaphragm
was more involved in the breathing process. During the 4-week period of
resistance breathing practice, the chest EMG for normal breathing
dropped 50%, indicating the diaphragm was indeed becoming the main
respiratory muscle.

In addition to the fact that the EMG fatigue testing is ideally suited to
biofeedback instrumentation, biofeedback itself plays an important part in

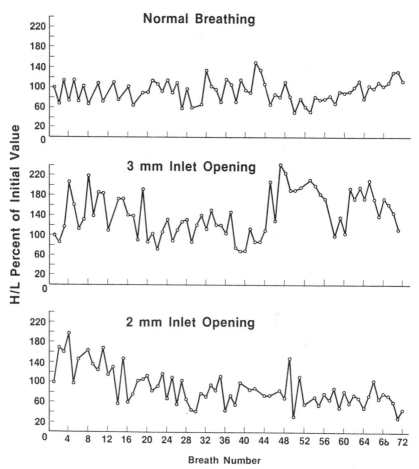

Fig 7–10.—The H/L ratio as a percent of initial value as a function of breath number for COLD patients. The top panel represents breathing through a valve with no resistance, and the middle and bottom panels represent resistance breathing.

inspiratory resistance breathing training. At the end of each inspiratory resistance breathing test, the patient is asked to rate his feeling on the 0 to 10 subjective feeling scale (Table 7–1) and 0 to 10 on the shortness of breath scale shown in Table 7–7. At the two extremes of the breathing scale, 0 indicates normal breathing and 10 is panic breathing. In many cases, it was found that for zero valve resistance (maximum inlet opening) the COLD patient reported tense feelings and mild shortness of breath. The mere act of putting on a nose clip and breathing through some kind of

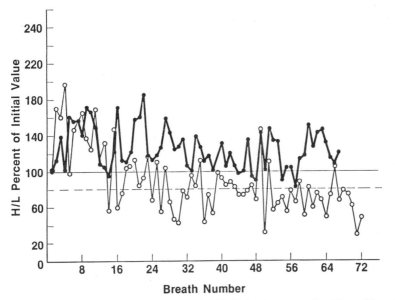

Fig 7–11.—The H/L ratio as a percent of initial value as a function of breath number while breathing against the lowest value of inlet opening (2 mm) sufficient to produce a decrease in H/L at the time of the initial measurements. The open circles represent pretraining data, and the closed circles represent post-training data after 4 weeks. The solid and dashed lines are for H/L ratios of 100% and 80% respectively.

a device was sufficient to produce shortness of breath. However, when they were instructed to use those principles learned in biofeedback and relax, they were then able to use the resistance device without becoming tense and short of breath. These observations further support the principle that there is a great deal of anxiety surrounding the breathing process itself for the COLD patient. This clinical observation shows the vital role that biofeedback plays in pulmonary rehabilitation.

TABLE 7–6.—INTEGRATED UPPER PECTORAL EMG FOR
INSPIRATORY RESISTANCE TEST (Figs 7–10 and 7–11)

DATE	UPPER PECTORAL EMG (μV)	INLET SIZE (mm)	FATIGUE INDICATED
12/9/82	2.53	–*	no
12/9/82	2.78	3	no
12/9/82	9.04	2	yes
1/4/83	3.07	2	no

*No restriction at inlet of valve.

TABLE 7–7.—INTENSITY OF
SHORTNESS OF BREATH SCALE

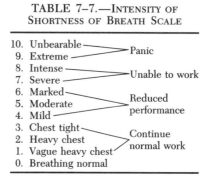

10. Unbearable
9. Extreme
8. Intense
7. Severe
6. Marked
5. Moderate
4. Mild
3. Chest tight
2. Heavy chest
1. Vague heavy chest
0. Breathing normal

Panic

Unable to work

Reduced
performance

Continue
normal work

Biofeedback For Weaning COLD Patients From Respirators

Patients with lung diseases have frequent respiratory crises that often require the mechanical support of ventilation. Certain types of patients may have prolonged weaning from assisted ventilation, and sometimes the weaning is extremely difficult. Corson and colleagues[30] presented two case studies in which patients were weaned from ventilators using biofeedback. However, before biofeedback is used to facilitate weaning, an EMG fatigue test[29] (described in the previous section) of the diaphragm and intercostal muscles should be made. The patient does not need to perform inspiratory resistance breathing, but the fatigue test is to determine if the diaphragm is fatiguing during normal breathing off the ventilator. The EMG fatigue test will help to determine whether the difficulty in weaning is due largely to muscle fatigue or anxiety and other psychological causes. If the diaphragm is fatiguing, then more emphasis should be given to rest periods after breathing off the respirator to ensure complete recovery from fatigue.

If there is no indication of diaphragm fatigue, then it is reasonable to conclude that difficulty in weaning is due to the fear and anxiety of not being able to breathe off the ventilator. In both of the case studies presented by Corson and coworkers,[30] the patients were given biofeedback. Tidal volume (VT) and respiration rate were used as feedback information. An oscilloscope was the feedback display device. The objects of the biofeedback were to increase VT and slow the respiratory rate. The sweep rate of the oscilloscope was set at a constant rate and the number of breaths per sweep successively lowered. In order to increase VT, two horizontal markers were placed on the oscilloscope. The distance between the markers reflected the target VT as the patient breathed more deeply. The amplitude of the oscilloscope tracing would increase, indicating greater VT. As the patient improved, the distance between the markers was increased to make the VT target slightly larger.

During biofeedback training, the patients achieved a larger V_T, which according to Corson and coworkers[30] resulted in exceeding the vital capacity (VC) of 10 ml/kg of body weight for successful weaning from the ventilator. They stated that the two case studies did not establish with certainty that increases in VC were due to biofeedback. However, evidence that biofeedback was an important factor in weaning was the rapid improvement in VC that occurred only after the start of biofeedback training.

Professional Qualifications for Performing Pulmonary Biofeedback

The above review shows that biofeedback performs a very important function in pulmonary rehabilitation. For the pulmonary patient, this means biofeedback aids in (1) a reduction in anxiety, (2) more ability to report feelings without getting short of breath, (3) improved breathing retraining, (4) inspiratory resistance breathing training and EMG fatigue testing, and (5) weaning from the ventilator as a result of respiratory crises. The above areas involve at least five health professional disciplines and, to some degree, psychology, physics, pulmonary medicine, respiratory therapy, physical therapy, and nursing. Psychologists have the necessary training for performing in the first two areas. Respiratory therapists are trained to perform nonbiofeedback functions in areas 3 through 5. Psychologists and, because of the complex physical measurements involved (particularly the EMG fatigue testing), even physicists have performed biofeedback in areas 3 and 4. However, because of the anxiety, fear, and other emotional factors underlying the above areas, as well as the need for patient management, it would seem more reasonable for the COLD patient to be treated with biofeedback under the direction of a psychologist who has some training in complex physical measurements in areas such as physics. The author of this chapter, for example, is licensed in the area of clinical psychology and has graduate training in both psychology and physics.

Regardless of which professionals perform biofeedback in areas 3 to 5, those professionals should be certified by the Biofeedback Certification Institute of America (BCIA). The purpose of the certification program is to provide a standard that health care professionals of all disciplines, the public, and other official groups accept as reliable evidence that a person has attained specified professional competency in biofeedback. It may seem a simple matter to purchase some biofeedback equipment, turn it on, and tell the person to relax his body. However, with any health care intervention there are hidden pitfalls of which a therapist needs to be aware in order to avoid harming the patient, and biofeedback is no exception to the rule. An individual certified in biofeedback by the BCIA is listed in a register of accredited specialists. This register is made available to all health organizations, consumer organizations, and insurance and medical groups. Certification will be important in insurance coverage for biofeedback therapy. Health professionals wishing certification may write to the BCIA address below for information:

Biofeedback Certification Institute of America
4301 Owens St.
Wheat Ridge, CO 80033
(303)420-2902

References

1. Jacobson E.: *Progressive Relaxation*. Chicago, University of Chicago Press, 1938.
2. Davis M.H., Saunders D.R., Greer T.L., Chai H.: Relaxation training facilitated by biofeedback apparatus as supplemental treatment in bronchial asthma. *J. Psychosom. Res.* 17:121-128, 1973.
3. Kotses H., Glaus K.D., Crawford P.L., et al.: Operant reduction of frontalis EMG activity in treatment of asthma in children. *J. Psychosom. Res.* 20:453–459, 1976.
4. Kotses H., Glaus K.D., Bricel S.K., et al.: Operant muscular reduction and peak expiratory flow rate in asthmatic children. *J. Psychosom. Res.* 22:17–23, 1978.
5. Kahn A.U., Staek M., Bonk C.: Role of counter-condition in the treatment of asthma. *J. Psychosom. Res.* 18:89–92, 1974.
6. Kahn A.U.: Effectiveness of biofeedback and counter-conditioning in the treatment of bronchial asthma. *J. Psychosom. Res.* 21:97–104, 1977.
7. Olton D.S., Noonberg, A.R.: *Biofeedback: Clinical Applications in Behavioral Medicine*. Englewood Cliffs, N.J. Prentice-Hall, Inc., 1980, pp. 221–251.
8. Kotses H., Glaus K.D.: Applications of biofeedback to the treatment of asthma: A critical review. *Biofeedback Self Regul.* 6:573–594, 1981.
9. Alexander A.B., Miklich D.R., Hershkoff H.: The immediate effects of systematic relaxation training on peak expiration flow rates in asthmatic children. *Psychosom. Med.* 34:388–394, 1972.
10. Alexander A.B., Grupp G.A., Chai H.: The effects of relaxation of pulmonary mechanics in children with asthma. *J. Appl. Behav. Anal.* 12:27–35, 1979.
11. Erskine J., Schonell M.: Relaxation therapy in bronchial asthma. *J. Psychosom. Res.* 23:121–134, 1979.
12. Holliday J.E., Munz D.: Changes in locus of control due to biofeedback, in Proceedings of Ninth Annual Meeting of the Biofeedback Society of America. Albuquerque, N.M., 1978.
13. Broussard R.: Using relaxation for COPD. *Am. J. Nurs.* 11:1962–1963, 1979.
14. Sitzman J.: Biofeedback for COPD Patients. *Occup. Health Nurs.* vol. 39, 1979.
15. Yanda R.L.: Biofeedback in pulmonary diseases. *West. J. Med.* 131:50–51, 1979.
16. Johnston R., Lee K.H.: Myofeedback: A new method of teaching breathing exercises in emphysematous patients. *Phys. Ther.* 56:826–831, 1976.
17. Dudley D.L., et al.: Psychosocial concomitants to rehabilitation in chronic obstructive pulmonary disease: I. Psychosocial and psychological considerations. *Chest* 77:413–420, 1980.

18. Dudley D.L., et al.: Psychosocial concomitants to rehabilitation in chronic obstructive pulmonary disease: II. Psychosocial treatment. *Chest* 77:544–551, 1980.
19. Hodgkin J.E., et al.: Chronic obstructive airway diseases. *J.A.M.A.* 232:1243–1260, 1975.
20. Holliday J.E., Ruppel G., McDaniels S.: Comparison of biofeedback emphysema patients and chronically anxious patients, in Proceedings of the Fourteenth Annual Meeting of the Biofeedback Society of America. Denver, 1983, pp. 107–110.
21. Miller C.: *Simultaneous Statistical Inference.* New York, McGraw-Hill Book Co., 1969.
22. Gaarder K.: Control of states of consciousness. *Arch. Gen. Psychiatry* 25:436–441, 1971.
23. Green E., et al.: Feedback technique for deep relaxation. *Psychophysiology* 6:371–377, 1969.
24. Basmajian J.V., Baeza M.D.., Fabrigar C.: Conscious control and training of individual spinal motor neurons in normal subjects. *J. New Drugs* 5:78–85, 1965.
25. James W.: *The Principles of Psychology.* Dover, N.Y., Henry Holt & Co., 1950.
26. Petty T.L., Hudson L.D., Neff T.A.: Methods of ambulatory care. *Med. Clin. North Am.* 57:751–761, 1973.
27. Basmajian J.V.: *Muscles Alive,* ed. 4. Baltimore, Williams & Wilkins Co., 1978.
28. Kaiser E., Petersen I.: Frequency analysis of muscle action potentials during tetanic contraction. *Electromyography* 3:5–17, 1963.
29. Gross D. et al.: The effect of training on strength and endurance of the diaphragm in quadriplegia. *Am. J. Med.* 68:27–35, 1980.
30. Corson J.A., et al.: Use of biofeedback in weaning paralysed patients from respirators. *Chest* 76:543–545, 1979.

8 / Oxygen Therapy

JERRY A. O'RYAN, B.S., R.R.T.

THIS CHAPTER ADDRESSES the physiologic rationale and subsequent ordering of oxygen therapy. Because an understanding of the pulmonary vascular bed and its normal anatomic and physiologic function is an important preliminary to discussing the alterations that lead to the need for oxygen therapy, a review of normal pulmonary vascular anatomy and physiology precedes the discussion of oxygen delivery systems.

Normal Pulmonary Vascular Anatomy and Physiology

The pulmonary arterial system consists of a gradual transition from the main pulmonary artery trunk to arterioles and then to capillaries. The pulmonary trunk, its bifurcating main pulmonary arteries, and the dichotomous extralobular pulmonary arteries are of an elastic consistency. Distinctive layers of elastic fibers embedded in a coat of muscle cells microscopically identify these arteries, whose external diameter is greater than 1,000 mμ.

The muscular pulmonary arteries are next, of a size ranging from 100 to 1,000 mμ. Found within lung lobules and paralleling bronchioles, these are morphologically identified by their thin medial layer of muscle tissue situated between elastic tissue. The pulmonary arterioles follow, with a range of 100 mμ or less. These vessels contain a partial layer of muscle that gradually lessens as the arteriole meets the pulmonary capillary dichotomy. Endothelial tissue elastic laminae are what remain of the arteriole prior to its connection with the pulmonary capillary bed.[1] Some gas exchange occurs at the distal end of these arterioles, as evidenced by postmortem studies on dogs, where well-oxygenated red blood cells (RBCs) were found at this point.[2]

The bulk of gas exchange, of course, takes place in the pulmonary capillary bed. These extremely thin-walled vessels are approximately 0.1 μ in external diameter. It is this ultra-thin lumen that allows only 75 to 100 ml of blood to serve the entire alveolar surface area of the lungs. The total pulmonary blood volume equals 500 ml. Single file RBCs pass through these microsized blood vessels. Conversely, in left heart failure (e.g., mitral stenosis as a dramatic situation), the resultant high-backup pressures may distend the capillaries enough to enable three to four RBCs to pass through side by side.[2]

Pulmonary Vascular Pressures

There are three pulmonary vascular pressure reference points to distinguish:[2]

1. *Absolute intravascular pressure* is the actual blood pressure (BP) in the lumen of any vessel at any point relative to atmospheric pressure.

2. *Transmural pressure* is the difference between the pressure in the lumen of a vessel and that of the tissue surrounding it. Intraluminal compliance is maintained by the fluid flowing through it. Extraluminal influences (i.e., surrounding tissues pressing against the vessel) tend to cause a compression on the vessel. The pressure on the pulmonary arteries and veins is caused by intrathoracic pressure; normally, the only extraluminal pressures exerted here are those caused by inspiration and expiration. Pressures around the arterioles, capillaries, and venules are due to a relative lessening effect of the alveolar and intrapleural pressures during quiet ventilation and in the absence of disease. Ventilatory maneuvers such as the Valsalva and Mueller maneuvers and coughing are evenly distributed throughout the thorax; thus no one particular area of the lungs and vasculature is singled out for any untoward target effect.[3]

3. *Driving pressure* is simply the difference in pressure from one point in a vessel when compared with another point downstream. Physically, it is a pressure gradient, and it is this gradient that is responsible for blood flow between these two points. Of course, blood viscosity and patency of the vessel lumen play a part in the net result of driving pressure. Total pulmonary circulation driving pressure is the difference between the pulmonary artery and the left atrium. Figure 8–1 gives an overall picture of the various pressures in relation to where the blood is flowing at any given anatomic point in the pulmonary and systemic circulatory system.

Pulmonary Artery Pressures in COLD

Pulmonary hypertension is said to exist when the systolic pulmonary BP is above 30 mm Hg and the diastolic pressure is above 15 mm Hg. In the absence of COLD, the pulmonary artery pressure does not rise very much, even during exercise. However, in the COLD patient whose disease has caused (1) loss of alveolar-capillary surface area along with (2) a concomitant hypoxemia, these factors account for an increased pulmonary artery pressure of greater than 30 mm Hg, often rising as high as 60 mm Hg or more. We will now look at the pathophysiology of these symptoms.

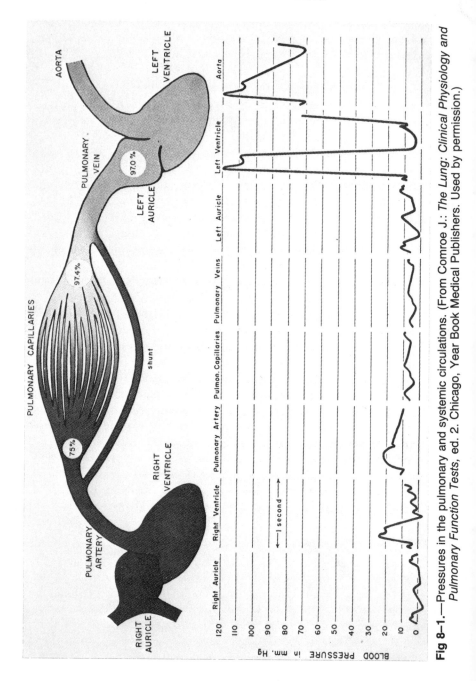

Fig 8–1.—Pressures in the pulmonary and systemic circulations. (From Comroe J.: *The Lung: Clinical Physiology and Pulmonary Function Tests*, ed. 2. Chicago, Year Book Medical Publishers. Used by permission.)

Pulmonary Hypertension

Prior to a discussion of oxygen therapy and its role in the pulmonary rehabilitation patient, there must be a comprehensive understanding of one of the primary factors leading to the need for oxygen in the ambulatory setting, *pulmonary hypertension*. Pulmonary hypertension may present as a chronic situation where it may be status quo for the severe COLD patient. It may also arise during periods of acute exacerbation, the onslaught and duration being somewhat inversely proportional to the aggressiveness of its treatment. Regardless of its clinical genesis and duration, the three main factors[4] precipitating and maintaining pulmonary hypertension are as follows:

1. *Decreased alveolar oxygen tension,* which causes a vasoconstrictive response to pulmonary vessels adjacent to alveoli with low P_{AO_2} levels. The result is a diversion of blood flow to alveoli with higher oxygen tensions.

2. *Decreased arterial oxygen tensions,* concomitant with #1 above. Current research data [5] suggest that chronically low levels stimulate vasoconstriction via a reflex action. Two such reflexes are thought to be smooth-muscle spasticity and release of chemical mediators because of the low oxygen tensions.

3. *Acidemia,* caused by low blood pH levels, which increases pulmonary vascular constriction. Chronic acidemia is a common precursor of acute pulmonary hypertension, and repeated episodes may lead to right heart failure.

Pathophysiology of Pulmonary Hypertension

The normal, nondiseased pulmonary vascular system previously described can usually accommodate the passive volume and pressure changes that occur in the lungs. It can usually compensate for even mild states of COLD without any untoward hypertensive reactions. It is the overt, consistent, and active stimulation occurring both systemically and locally that creates the increased volumes and pressures regarded to be of a clinical hypertensive quality.

The two stimuli cited most often as precipitators of chronic pulmonary hypertension are *hypoxia* and *acidosis*.[4-7] Hypoxia will be discussed first, because it is thought to be the greater of the two stimulants.

Systemically, hypoxemia causes the carotid body receptors to trigger a systemic arteriolar vasoconstriction.[6] Locally and more importantly, hypoxemia causes a vasoconstrictive response in the pulmonary arteries and arterioles via two methods: (1) an *indirect* method, wherein alveolar hypoxia supposedly causes certain cells (e.g., mast cells) in the pulmonary parenchyma to release vasoactive substances such as histamine, which causes a localized vasoconstrictive response, or (2) a *direct* constrictive response on the smooth muscles of the pulmonary vessel walls.[5] The actual mechanism of the latter is not known, but it is believed to be the result of a direct effect of low Pa_{O_2} on the walls of the resistance vessels of the lung. Figure 8–2 illustrates these two mechanisms. Fraser and associates[6] delineate the direct vasoconstrictive response even more by suggesting that the vasoconstrictive site of action is perhaps on the arteriole that accompanies the terminal bronchiole, i.e., the arteriole that supplies circulation to the acinar unit.

Acidosis is considered to be the next most powerful stimulant causing pulmonary hypertension, mainly because of its pressor effect on the pulmonary circulation. It also reinforces the hypoxic stimulant for a net synergistic effect. The blood pH levels, as opposed to elevated P_{CO_2} levels, give rise to this response, because hypercapnic patients can usually compensate for higher P_{CO_2} levels by increasing their minute ventilation to maintain near normal CO_2 levels in the blood.[5] Another source of acidotic

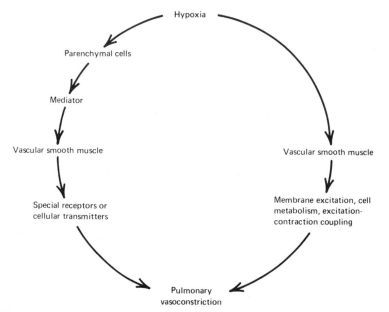

Fig 8–2.—Alternative mechanisms of action of hypoxia. Alveolar hypoxia causes cells in the pulmonary parenchyma to release vasoactive substances (left pathway), or hypoxia (by alveoli or blood) acts directly on pulmonary vascular smooth muscle to elicit vasoconstriction (right pathway). (From Fishman A.P.: *Pulmonary Diseases and Disorders,* vol. 1. New York, McGraw-Hill Book Co., 1980. Used by permission.)

stimulation is at the tissue level. The cellular hypoxia causes the normal oxidative phosphorylation system (aerobic system) to shift to an energy-producing system that functions anaerobically. This metabolic shift causes an increase in lactate and lactic acid, which then leads to a metabolic acidosis. The end result at the lung level is an additive effect of even more vasoconstriction precipitated by the low pH levels.[8]

Other Organ Responses to Chronic Hypoxemia

Less data are available on other organs' responses to chronic hypoxemia. A brief summary is given here to at least acquaint the practitioner with those responses.

Acute hypoxemia occurring when the patient has an exacerbation crisis produces a variety of cardiac arrhythmias, most notably ST segment depression. This is more likely to occur during periods of heavy exercise. In the clinic, it is even likely to show up under a supervised activity such as treadmill exercise. Chronic effects include right ventricular hypertrophy.[8] Sustained mean pulmonary artery pressures above 40 mm Hg are usually considered to be a good indication of possible right ventricular hypertrophy. Radiographs and ECGs help to bear this out when suspected.[9]

Cerebral responses to chronic hypoxemia are manifested by decelerated mentation, vertigo, decreased psychomotor coordination, initial restlessness, headache, and other symptoms. An excellent study by Krop and co-workers showed that low-flow oxygen therapy improved those deficits of a cognitive nature (e.g., mentation).

Renal function in chronic hypoxemia is paradoxic; that is, mild degrees

TABLE 8–1.—EFFECTS OF CHRONIC HYPOXEMIA ON THE BODY ORGANS

PULMONARY	CARDIAC	CEREBRAL	RENAL
(−) Constricts pulmonary vessels	(−) Right ventricular hypertrophy	(−) Decreases mentation, coordination, visual activity, reaction time	(−) Decreases blood flow (severe hypoxemia)
(−) Raises mean pulmonary artery pressure	(*) Increased pulse rate	(*) Dilates vessels	(+) Increases blood flow (mild hypoxemia)
(+) Decreases shunts in low ventilating alveoli	(*) Increased cardiac output	(−) transient ischemic attacks	(*) Stimulates erythropoietin to increase RBC production
		(−) Insomnia	
		(−) Restlessness	

(−) Negative response.
(+) Relatively positive response.
(*) Positive response at first, then long-term effects are negated, usually resulting in further pathology and clinical symptoms.

of hypoxemia (Pa_{O_2} greater than 40 mm Hg) increases renal function. A study by Kilburn and colleagues[11] reports in depth on the effects of hypoxia, hyperoxia, and hypercapnia on renal function.

Table 8–1 lists the general organ responses to chronic hypoxemia.

Patient Selection For Oxygen Therapy

The baseline rationale for oxygen therapy is that it should be used when severe persistent hypoxemia persists after all other hospital modalities have failed to correct the problem (e.g., cardiac stabilization, reversal and maintenance of bronchospasm, bronchopulmonary hygiene measures, nutrition levels, and so on).

In addition to persistent marked hypoxemia (after the above measures have been taken), the patient may also exhibit some or all of the following symptoms:

1. Severe dyspnea on moderate-to-heavy exercise disproportionate to pulmonary mechanics

2. Persistent and recurring congestive heart failure (CHF) uncorrected by usual cardiotonic measures

3. Severe, recurring erythrocytosis

4. Decreased mentation and behavioral changes

5. Restlessness

6. Severe hypoxemia nocturnally as evidenced by ear oximetry studies

The American Thoracic Society officially recommended the following as indications for long-term oxygen therapy:[12]

1. Evidence of reduced mixed venous oxygen (primary factor)

2. Pulmonary hypertension

3. Cor pulmonale

4. Increasing severity of hypoxemia with exercise

5. Exercise limited by hypoxia, but relieved by oxygen

6. Polycythemia

In a report from the American College of Chest Physicians in 1973,[8] the following observation was made: "The aim of oxygen therapy in ambulatory patients with chronic obstructive lung disease is to overcome tissue hypoxia; it is usually necessary only to *improve* hypoxemia rather than correct it completely." Thus, some portion of hypoxemic ventilatory drive may be retained while minimizing the worsening of hypercapnia that could occur from oxygen therapy. Additionally, long-term survival is not threatened by the possibility of oxygen toxicity[13]; therefore, the prescriber should not be concerned about continuous low-flow oxygen effects on the alveolar tissue in regard to an increased mortality rate from toxic oxygen effects.

Fox and Snider[14] suggest the following general guidelines for patient selection when prescribing oxygen in the ambulatory setting:

1. Hypoxemia persists after an active treatment program using *all other* methods of respiratory care.
2. One or more signs or symptoms of hypoxemia are present:
   a. Chronic cor pulmonale, especially with right heart failure
   b. Erythrocytosis with a hematocrit greater than 55%
   c. Severe dyspnea upon exercise with resultant fatigue and falling Pa_{O_2}
   d. Impairment of cognitive functions
   e. Sleep disturbances
3. All patients with resting Pa_{O_2} levels of less than 45 mm Hg (mandatory) and oxygen should be considered in patients with Pa_{O_2} levels 45 to 55 mm Hg.

Until the publication of the initial Nocturnal Oxygen Therapy Trial (NOTT),[15] patient selection and oxygen dosages/durations expected to be used by the patient appeared to be somewhat random. Early articles in which the authors discuss their selection of patients and oxygen dosages varies. (The reader is directed to review articles dealing with low-flow oxygen therapy prior to 1974, especially those appearing before 1970. A complete list is not given here because of space considerations.) One of the earlier references suggesting a nocturnal oxygen vs. continuous oxygen therapy trial was by Block in 1974.[7] However, as early as 1968, studies were being done to determine the effects of long-term oxygen therapy. In one such study, Abraham and colleagues[16] studied the effects of continuous oxygen in a 4- to 8-week duration on six patients. Their results showed a gradual fall in pulmonary artery pressure; the mean pressure for the group was 42.5 mm Hg before and 32.3 mm Hg after the study. Hematocrits decreased from a mean of 51.4% to 42.5%. Other studies basically confirmed the same results.[17-19]

Objectives of Oxygen Therapy

The main objective of continuous low-flow oxygen is to maintain the patient's resting blood oxygen level at 55 to 60 mm Hg and exercise levels at a level of 50 mm Hg. The hypoxic respiratory drive is thought to be stimulated at a Pa_{O_2} of 60 mm Hg or less.

It is important to realize that we are not attempting to return the patient's blood oxygen levels to those found in a person in a nonpulmonary disease state, i.e., a Pa_{O_2} of 80 to 100 mm Hg. The HbO_2 saturation curve does not demand this high of a Pa_{O_2} for adequate saturation. Also, the very real likelihood of a decreased ventilatory drive may result in those patients whose Pa_{O_2} have been injudiciously elevated. It must be remembered that COLD patients, especially those with chronically high P_{CO_2} levels, no longer are stimulated to breathe by central P_{CO_2} chemoreceptor stimulation, but instead by a peripheral chemoreceptor hypoxic drive. Overoxygenation of patients with chronic compensated CO_2 retention, and who are thus breathing because of a hypoxic drive, must be warned not to turn their oxygen up and down on a mere whim or because of sudden subjective feelings of dyspnea. Instead, blood gas analysis or ear oxygen saturation studies should dictate the patient's actual oxygen requirements.

Obviously, the actual oxygen requirements will vary from patient to patient. However, the objectives of prescribing oxygen therapy in COLD patients, whether for continuous or intermittent use, differ from those in the nondiseased patient. The major difference, of course, is that the use of oxygen in the nondiseased patient is for a one-time use or for a relatively short duration, with the prime objective being to purposely elevate the patient's Pa_{O_2} to normal physiologic levels. Also, there are usually no permanent alterations to the patient's acid-base, hematologic, neurologic, and general organ oxygen-dependent status because of the virtue of the short-lived hypoxic crisis—assuming, of course, that oxygen was administered in a timely fashion. However, the subtle, slow pathologic changes of COLD allow for these physiologic and anatomic changes to occur over such a long period of time that usually the patient is not overtly aware of them until his first exacerbation occurs. It is at this time that the true clinical picture of COLD is seen and a quantitative diagnosis made. The point is that it is the very chronicity of the lung disease and associated body response changes (as opposed to one-time, acute hypoxic crisis in otherwise normal individuals with an expected 100% reversal of the symptoms) that delineate the objectives for prescribing oxygen in COLD patients. In other words, this is why we use a different set of objectives when prescribing oxygen for long-term use whether continuous or intermittent. Shapiro and associates state: "The general principle of 'minimal' oxygen administration consistent with adequate cardiopulmonary homeostasis always holds true!"[4] This principle should be the guiding tenet, especially for COLD patients receiving continuous oxygen therapy. Following are objectives to keep in mind when prescribing oxygen for COLD patients in the ambulatory setting:

1. To relieve dyspnea while at rest or with mild exercise.
2. To maintain oxygen saturation levels at 80% +.
3. To reduce pulmonary hypertension.
4. To prevent cardiomegaly due to chronic hypoxemia.
5. To maintain other nonpulmonary organs in a state of relative homeostasis.

Most severe COLD patients require oxygen at 1 to 2 L/min. *at least* 15 to 18 hours a day. Continuous oxygen (i.e., approaching 24 hours a day with some time allowed off for personal and hygienic considerations) is *best*. The initial NOTT study supports this dictum.[15]

Duration of total time may vary depending on the severity of the patient's hypoxemia as determined by initial baseline studies. An adequate synopsis of the initial NOTT study could not be done justice here, and the reader is encouraged to study the initial NOTT study and subsequent papers on it for a more comprehensive and updated understanding.

The reader may, of course, desire a pat answer regarding *exactly* how much and how long the patient should be on oxygen therapy. There is no formula per se to allow us to extract those answers. The severity of the patient's disease and resultant secondary pathologies will determine longevity of oxygen usage. Again, the reader is referred to the list above for review, because it suggests the criteria that the practitioner should use when prescribing and following the patient's clinical course. (Chapter 2 also details the methods used in evaluating the patient's response to oxygen therapy.)

Oxygen Delivery Systems

The premise for the prescription and use of oxygen for the pulmonary rehabilitation patient may at first appear to be simply an extension of in-hospital practices into the ambulatory setting. While the basic principle remains the same, i.e., to relieve hypoxemia, the actual ordering by the physician and subsequent daily use by the patient does not parallel the same rationale as ordering oxygen for the hospitalized patient. A very pragmatic example illustrates: When ordering oxygen for the inpatient, it is taken for granted that the oxygen is already there, literally, merely waiting on the other side of a wall outlet. Ordering oxygen for the ambulating or even bedbound outpatient involves quite a bit more forethought and preparation as the following list of considerations indicates:

1. What type of system should be ordered (cylinder, liquid, or concentrator)?

2. How much instruction and follow-up care will the patient require in order to learn how to effectively and efficiently use his oxygen?

3. What oxygen supplier will be able to supply not only the best service, ensuring an uninterrupted supply of oxygen to the patient, but also be capable of catering to any specific oxygen-related needs of the patient?

4. How will the in-home use of the patient's oxygen and service by the oxygen supplier be monitored?

This section addresses all the above concerns and gives the reader a few other areas to consider and scrutinize.

Cylinder, Liquid, and Concentrator

The three oxygen delivery systems most commonly used in the ambulatory setting are (1) the time-honored high-pressure cylinder (2) liquid oxygen and (3) the oxygen concentrator (Fig 8–3). The rationale and guidelines for selecting the correct system for home-care oxygen delivery will be dis-

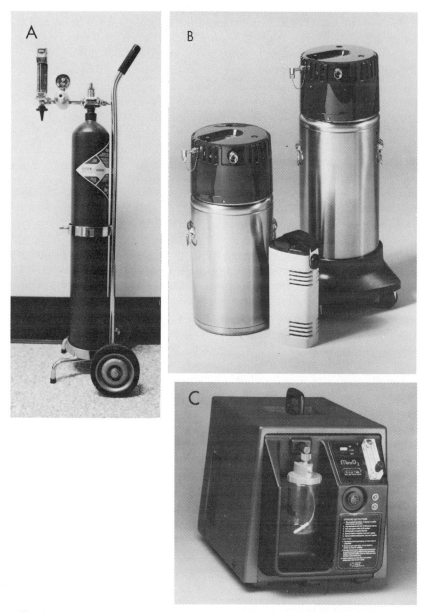

Fig 8–3.—A, E cylinder of oxygen. **B,** liquid oxygen (courtesy of Cryogenic Association, Indianapolis). **C,** oxygen concentrator (courtesy of Mountain Medical Equipment, Inc., Littleton, Colo.).

cussed. Responsibilities of both the prescribing physician and the oxygen supplier are also delineated. (Chapter 13 discusses these and other home-care guidelines in depth.)

A synopsis of the three oxygen delivery systems is given below. This chapter will not provide detailed technical information on the systems; this information is readily available from the manufacturers and home-care companies providing these units. However, as a point of reference, a brief description is given here.

1. *High-pressure oxygen cylinders.* These contain gaseous oxygen ready for immediate use. When a pressure reduction valve is turned, a flowmeter attached to the pressure gauge then meters out the gas in L/min. No alarms are on the cylinder to warn of failure or decreased pressure. A dial on the pressure gauge records remaining contents in pounds per square inch gauge (psig). The concentration of the gas is relatively 100%.

2. *Liquid oxygen systems.* Liquid oxygen stored at $-297°$ F in a thermos-like container is vaporized to a gaseous state continuously and passes out of the container as conventional, ready-to-use, therapeutic-quality oxygen at a concentration of relatively 100%.

Two units are used. One is a large 20-or 30-L reservoir container that can be used in the home and serves as a source for refilling the smaller tote-along system for use outside the home. The smaller unit contains enough liquid oxygen to supply the patient with 1 to 2 L/min for approximately 6 to 8 hours and weighs approximately 9½ lb.

3. *Oxygen concentrator.* This is a unique method of supplying therapeutic oxygen, because the self-contained unit performs this function on-site. Using what the manufacturers call a Molecular Sieve Pressure Swing Absorption (PSA) process, oxygen is separated from nitrogen and trace gases. The concentration decreases at proportionately higher flows: e.g., 93% at 0 to 2 L, 85% at 3 L, 80% at 4 L, and 70% at 6 L.[20]

There should not be a concern over these proportionately lower concentrations because most continuous oxygen therapy users only require low-flow rates, besides which the objective is only to raise the inspired oxygen level (FI_{O_2}) to 24% to 40% in most cases in order to achieve Pa_{O_2} levels of 55 to 60 mm Hg.

All three systems can be used with conventional permanent or disposable humidifiers. Figure 8–4 suggests which system may be of optimal benefit cost-wise, based on daily usage. Table 8–2 lists the benefits and limitations of the three oxygen delivery systems just discussed.

Guidelines for Prescribing Home Oxygen Systems

All three systems have their usefulness and appropriateness for the ambulatory or semiambulatory patient. It is the amount of patient mobility

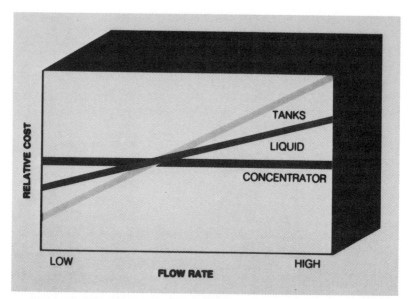

Fig 8–4.—Cost comparisons. Cost-effectiveness of a particular method depends primarily on the quality of oxygen used over a given period of time. Tanks and liquid systems are usually less expensive at low usage rates (low flows and/ or limited periods of use). The cost of a concentrator remains the same regardless of use. Therefore, concentrators are usually more cost-effective in the mid to high usage ranges. (Courtesy of Mountain Medical Equipment, Inc., Littleton, Colo.)

and daily expected duration of oxygen usage which serves as the decision-making basis for which system or combination of systems will work best for the patient. The prescribing physician and therapist/home-care coordinator should keep the following guidelines in mind when ordering oxygen for home use:

1. *Current and future anticipated mobility of the patient.* Here, one must look at the patient's current domestic work and social lifestyle. A more mobile system such as a portable liquid system would be indicated for the patient still able to enjoy outside activities.

2. *Requirements of the relatively home-bound patient.* A portable liquid system may not be efficacious, both practically speaking and cost-wise, when the user is essentially confined to the home with only intermittent short excursions outside. The higher cost of the liquid system and the inherent evaporation action of its content, whether in use or not, needs to be considered as a cost liability for this patient. A concentrator with an E-size high-pressure cylinder for excursions outside the home may be more practical and cost-beneficial.

TABLE 8–2.—A COMPARISON OF BENEFITS AND LIMITATIONS OF OXYGEN DELIVERY SYSTEMS

	CONVENTIONAL HIGH-PRESSURE CYLINDERS	LIQUID OXYGEN	OXYGEN CONCENTRATORS
BENEFITS	Ready to use	Both reservoir and portable units provide large amounts of O_2 in relatively small containers	Least expensive system if used 18 hr or more per day at low flows; 12 hr at higher flows (relative hours and flows)
	100% concentration	No outside maintenance normally required	No refilling needed
	No maintenance required	No noise except for hissing as pressure relief activates	Few mechanical problems on newer models
	No noise	Portable unit fairly easily handled without tiring patient	New smaller models easy to move around; takes up little space
	Can provide high flows if needed	Can provide adequate flows up to 6 L/min (most units) if needed	Aesthetically pleasing due to furniture-like design
LIMITATIONS	High users must have constant refills weekly; takes up much storage space	High users must have refills up to twice weekly	High concentrations of oxygen not available when rates flow exceed 6 L/min
	Potential safety-handling problems	Non-ambidextrous patients may have trouble refilling small unit off reservoir	Must be checked periodically; filters must be cleaned
	Large cylinders very heavy; difficult to move with ease	Expense can be very high for continuous oxygen users	Must have large cylinder backup in case of unit or electric power failure
			Large older models bulky, noisy

3. *Requirements of the COLD patient whose mobility is severely limited.*
Again, a concentrator may be the best answer to this patient's needs. A
patient who is severely disabled and essentially bedfast requiring continuous low-flow oxygen, will find a liquid system very costly, and because
mobility may not be an expected goal of the patient (i.e., terminal cancer
or end-stage COLD), the virtues of portable oxygen are not a consideration
here. A high-pressure M-, G-, or H-size cylinder should also be provided
with the concentrator in case of unit or electrical power failure.

In summary, the objective of prescribing the right system(s) for the right
patient involves careful scrutiny of his needs with an optimistic allowance
for hopefully continued ambulation and mild exercise relative to the severity of his disease state. See Appendix A for calculating F_{IO_2}.

The Nasal Cannula

Undoubtedly the most widely used appliance for actual delivery of the
oxygen to the patient, the cannula does pose its own inherent problems.
Besides irritation of the nares, discomfort to the top of the ears is a problem. The following article reprint shows how two patients, working independently, came up with two separate and ingenious methods of alleviating
the problem of ear discomfort. The method by which the two patients devised their "cannula comforters" is described below.

New Comfort for Nasal Cannula Users*

The nasal cannula is one of the most widely used means of delivering low flow
oxygen. It is simple, safe and reliable. It is convenient in that it allows the patient
to speak and eat while receiving continuous oxygen therapy. The nasal cannula has
been shown to be effective in those patients classified as "mouth breathers."

One of the few drawbacks of this device is the discomfort sometimes felt on the
top of the ears, especially when worn continuously. However, Mr. Foryst Winship
and Mr. Richard Davis have each come up with an ingenious way to deal with this
problem.

Mr. Winship has been on continuous home oxygen for four years. As a result of
wearing eyeglasses and wearing a nasal cannula continuously, his ears had become
a nearly constant source of pain. However, about 6 months ago, he came upon the
idea of attaching a rubber band from a button on his shirt to his nasal cannula in
such a manner that it would support the weight of the oxygen tube. As a result,
very little pressure would be applied to his ears. This worked well in some situations, such as when he was sitting, but he soon found he needed something a bit
more sturdy. Based on his original idea, he soon invented Winship's Cannula Support Necklace (Fig 8–5).

This consists of little more than a 24-inch shoelace and the plastic cap of a medicine bottle. The cap should have three holes in it, specifically one in the center

*Reprinted from Mays M.K.: New comfort for nasal cannula users. *J. Ventilation* 10:7,
1982. Copyright 1982, Ohio Society for Respiratory Therapy. Used by permission.

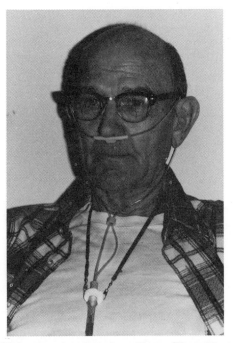

Fig 8–5.—Winship's cannula support necklace. (From Mays M.K.: New comfort for nasal cannula users. *J. Ventilation* 10:7, 1982. Used by permission.)

about ¼ inch in diameter and a smaller one on either side just large enough to pull the shoelace through. The B & F Nasal Cannula Model #64208 (B & F Medical Products, Inc., 1421 Expressway Drive North, Toledo, Ohio), is ideally suited for use with this device as a result of the design of its tubing connector. To use the cannula support necklace, first push the cap over the end of the tubing connector on the cannula, then attach the cannula to the oxygen supply tubing. Then place the shoelace around the neck and pull either end through the two small holes far enough so that most of the weight of the tubing and cannula is supported by the shoelace, not the ears.

Mr. Richard Davis has been using oxygen at home for about two years. He, too, is a near continuous user and as a result had suffered with sore ears for quite some time. Over the years, Mr. Davis has enjoyed golfing, and during that time he had accumulated several sun visors. He solved his cannula problem by altering one as is shown below (Fig 8–6). He simply removed the bill and made his visor into a sweatband (which would work just as well) and attached a paper clip on either side just above the ears. He then bent the inner loop of the paper clip out to form a hook on which the cannula rests.

Both of these devices are ideally suited for home use in that they are easy to use and easy to make at home. However, either of them could also be well utilized in a hospital setting.

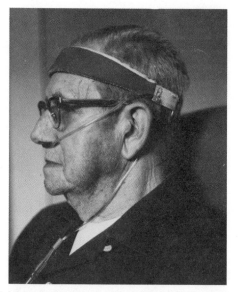

Fig 8–6.—Davis' headband hook. (From Mays M.K.: New comfort for nasal cannula users. *J. Ventilation* 10:7, 1982. Used by permission.)

Working with Home-Care Oxygen Vendors

The professional home-care oxygen and equipment company can be of great assistance in helping the prescriber of the oxygen to ensure that the right equipment is supplied. The vendor has only the prescriber's information to direct him when setting up oxygen for home use. Therefore, the prescriber had a dual obligation (to the patient and to the vendor) to be as concise as possible when writing orders for use of oxygen in the home.

After careful consideration of the previous guidelines, the prescriber needs to include the following information on the orders for home oxygen:

1. Diagnosis, including current arterial blood gas level, with any secondary complications

2. Type of system or combination of systems (e.g., concentrator with E cylinder).

3. Dosage in L/min.

4. How oxygen is to be inspired (e.g., cannula, face mask, etc.).

5. Expected duration of time patient will be on system per day (e.g., 12 hours, 15 hours, 18 to 24 hours).

6. Approximate total time patient is expected to use the system(s) (weeks, months, lifetime).

7. Anecdotal information may be verbalized, such as patient's mentation,

comprehension level, availability of family or neighbors' assistance, acceptance and attitude of patient toward his disease state, any psychomotor deficit that would restrict the patient in using the system, etc. Type of insurance and prior approval by the third-party payer is also gratefully acknowledged by the vendors.

A professional home-care supplier should be capable of doing and/or providing the following:

1. The vendor should be able to comprehend and follow through with your orders. Any deviations or allowances should be brought to your attention at the time of the initial order or as the occasion arises.

2. A competent and thorough explanation of the use, care, and safety of the system and any ancillary supplies to the patient is mandatory. The best trained person on the company's staff should do all initial setups and follow through at agreed-on time intervals. Of course, most systems will require either periodic refilling (cylinder and liquid oxygen) or intermittent preventative maintenance (oxygen concentrators). Many companies are now using credentialed, clinically active respiratory therapists for this area of responsibility. *Under no circumstance is there any excuse for a trained or untrained person to simply drop off the equipment with a simple explanation of "read the instructions"!*

3. Initial setup and monthly or preagreed-on time interval reports to the physician, respiratory therapist, and other professional interested parties should be written. This report should reiterate what the patient is using as well as anecdotal notations (see Tables 8–3 and 8–4).

4. If problems arise regarding the patient's compliance or use of equip-

TABLE 8–3.—Sample of Initial Equipment Set-Up Report

PATIENT: C.W.
          Miami Valley Hospital
          Dayton, Ohio
EQUIPMENT: "Mini-O_2" Oxygen Concentrator

Mrs. W.'s oxygen concentrator was set up in her home at 82 Elm St., Dayton, Ohio, on 7/5/82. Because she was still in the hospital, a return visit was made upon her arrival home on 7/5/82.

The concentrator and H-cylinder backup system were set up in the bedroom where she will be spending the majority of her time. A sufficient amount of tubing was used to permit the patient to reach both the bathroom and the kitchen. Because the patient lives alone and must do her own cooking, she was repeatedly instructed not to use the oxygen while cooking.

Mrs. W. was instructed on all aspects of operating and maintaining the oxygen concentrator and H-cylinder. Return demonstrations by Mrs. W. proved satisfactory.

A return visit will be made in a few days to assure the safe and proper use of the equipment and to answer any questions the patient may have.

This concludes our initial evaluation. You will be receiving a monthly report hereafter on this patient.

Signed

TABLE 8–4.—SAMPLE OF MONTHLY FOLLOW-UP REPORT

PATIENT: C.W.
      Miami Valley Hospital
      Dayton, Ohio
EQUIPMENT: "Mini-O_2"Oxygen Concentrator
SET-UP DATE: 7/5/82
    This is the monthly follow-up report for Mrs. W., made 8/6/82.
    We should first mention that a visit was made on 8/3/82 following a phone call from Mrs. W. She was very anxious and concerned that there was no flow coming through the cannula. We immediately visited the patient and found the unit to be functioning properly, with no alarms sounding and an oxygen concentration of 92% at 2 L/min. We demonstrated to the patient how to submerge the nosepiece in a clear glass of water to determine flow through the tubing.
    As we talked with Mrs. W., it was discovered that she was unable to routinely clean the humidifier bottle and air intake filters. There was no mention of this or of any difficulty with the concentrator during routine phone calls earlier in the month. We immediately made arrangements with the visiting homemaker and with a neighbor to help with the maintenance of the concentrator.
    During our follow-up visit a few days later, the "Mini-O_2" concentrator was functioning properly with an oxygen concentration of 94% at 2 L/min. The air intake filters were found to be clean and the humidifier properly filled with boiled distilled water. Routine replacement of the source gas inlet filters and adjustment of the pressure compensator was also performed. Since the visiting homemaker was present during our visit, we reviewed the proper technique for cleaning the humidifier bottles and filters.
    Mrs. W. complained of an infrequent cough with a slight amount of white sputum production. Her respiratory rate was 22/min, and her cardiac rate was 78 beats per minute. She stated she only felt dyspneic when she became upset or frustrated. She cited examples of forgetting where she put things or not being able to perform small tasks such as adding water to the humidifier bottle. She was instructed to call us whenever she had difficulties with the concentrator, no matter how small, as this is preferred to her becoming upset and, therefore, short of breath.
    Because Mrs. W. lives alone and has trouble ambulating, we will increase our calls and follow her progress more closely. Thank you for allowing us to assist this patient with her home-care needs.
Signed

ment, the home-care company representative should immediately inform the physician and others involved with the patient's care. The home-care and/or hospital-based pulmonary rehabilitation respiratory therapist is usually delegated the role of supervising the patient's home care and thus may be the usual source of communication when problems occur. It can then be the therapist's responsibility to contact the physician. Of course, all matters of a direct medical concern should be brought immediately to the physician's attention.

Transtracheal Oxygen[21–23]

A lightweight, completely portable transtracheal oxygen system that delivers oxygen directly into the lungs looks promising as an alternative to some current bulky oxygen delivery systems. The transtracheal oxygen concept works by inserting a No. 16 Teflon® catheter between the second and third tracheal rings (see Fig 8–7). Because oxygen is delivered directly to the tracheobronchial tree, bypassing the large anatomic deadspace of the upper airway, much lower flows of oxygen can be used. Flows as low as 0.25 to 1.5 L/min are possible.

Devised by Henry J. Heimlich, M.D. (developer of the Heimlich maneuver), the system allows a sharp reduction in oxygen usage, especially for continuous oxygen users who may use 2 to 4 L/min. The initial results have been very promising, and early studies of 14 patients show the greater majority not only tolerating the lower flows, but also ambulating much more, some even returning to work or enjoying higher levels of domestic activities.

The main advantages of transtracheal oxygen are best delineated when contrasted with the conventionally used nasal cannula. The latter has these drawbacks:

1. Waste factor is present because of anatomic deadspace.

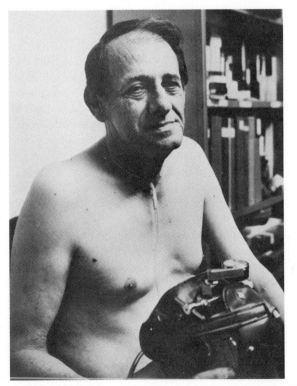

Fig 8–7.—Transtracheal oxygen. (Courtesy of H.J. Heimlich, M.D., Cincinnati.)

2. Higher liter flows are thus used, necessitating a readily accessible bulk supply of oxygen at all times.

3. The nasal cannula (and other nasofacial devices used, e.g., mask) require a long tubing to connect the patient's appliance to the oxygen delivery system, resulting in a physical (and psychological) tether to the system, which usually must be toted along with the patient.

4. Oxygen delivered through the nose or mouth tends to dry the nasopharyngeal mucosa, resulting in irritation and allergenic skin reactions at the nares in some patients and even bleeding erosions in a few cases.

5. An aesthetic aversion in some patients.

Heimlich's transtracheal oxygen system supposedly avoids all these drawbacks of conventionally delivered nasofacial oxygen by bypassing the whole upper airway. Other advantages of transtracheal oxygen include the following:

1. Less ventilatory effort is required to draw oxygen into the lungs, because oxygen enters directly at the tracheal site.

2. Oxygen delivery is not impaired by sinusitis, mouth breathing, cannula displacement, or loss of oxygen into the room.

3. Nutrition may improve, because oxygen supply is not interrupted while the patient is eating.

A very definite advantage of transtracheal oxygen to the budget-minded patient is the reduced costs of oxygen usage. Before-and after-placement analysis of oxygen consumption and related costs of a transtracheal oxygen catheter system shows a substantial decrease in the amount of oxygen used. For example, one patient's oxygen costs per month went from $410 to $146, a 64% cost reduction. Concomitantly, the same patient had earlier experienced a 19-week hospitalization for severe respiratory failure at a cost of approximately $33,000 prior to his transtracheal oxygen catheter insertion. In the first 1½ years after placement, this patient was not hospitalized for any pulmonary or related conditions. Finally, medication dosages (and thus costs) may decrease. Drugs such as bronchodilators, Digoxin, Lanoxin, Lasix, and prednisone, usually prescribed for hypoxemic-related problems, can be gradually decreased.

It is this author's opinion that we may expect to see the advent of transtracheal oxygen in the near future as a specially selected procedure, at least for oxygen administration in long-term, continuous oxygen users. However, more research and clinical work need to be performed.

Summary

The use of oxygen on a continuous basis for the chronic hypoxemic patient has proved to be of definite benefit. The NOTT study not only apprised health-care practitioners of the benefits of oxygen therapy, but also gave them an excellent initial data base from which further clinical research can be performed with resulting clinical applications. Future editions of this book will report those discoveries and resultant clinical uses.

A brief review of normal and disease-state anatomy and physiology showed that the primary site and most severely offended area resulting from COLD and hypoxemia is the pulmonary vasculature. The specific response to this is pulmonary hypertension. Long-term continuous oxygen therapy tends to decrease, though not totally reverse, this condition. Other symptoms include decreased cerebral responses, reduced renal outflow in severe hypoxemia, and right-heart hypertrophy and failure. These symptoms, too, are partially reversed by continuous oxygen administration.

When prescribing oxygen, the various systems (cylinder, liquid, and concentrator) must be considered in view of the patient's daily needs and the benefits/limitations each of these systems offers. An open and professional rapport between the prescribing physician, therapist, and home-care oxygen supplier is desirable in order to provide an oxygen delivery system and follow-up care that this type of patient sorely needs. Expedition and close tolerance of the physician's orders is gained when the physician and therapist carefully scrutinize the patient's at-home oxygen needs. The vendor has a responsibility to provide only well-trained personnel in the initial setup and subsequent visits.

What does the future hold for oxygen therapy delivery techniques? Refinement of the concentrator to one that is smaller and more portable has already been made. Within 3 to 5 years, a battery-powered, portable concentrator unit will probably be available in the range of 15 to 20 lbs or less.

Dr. Henry J. Heimlich has innovated a new method of delivering oxygen transtracheally.[21-23] An opening to permit a 12- to 16-gauge catheter is made between the second and third tracheal ring. Oxygen flows as small as one tenth the amount of nasally required oxygen may provide sufficient oxygen levels in the blood. Oxygen is provided by a 6-lb gaseous container. The virtues of the system at this time appear to be (1) smaller increments of oxygen to maintain acceptable Pa_{O_2} and (2) a more aesthetic approach to using oxygen. While more studies on this system are in order, it appears to be a promising advance in the field of oxygen therapy.

References

1. Murray J.F.: *The Normal Lung*. Philadelphia, W.B. Saunders Co., 1976.
2. Comroe J.H.: *Physiology of Respiration*. Chicago, Yearbook Medical Publishers, 1971.
3. Slonim N.B., Hamilton L.H.: *Respiratory Physiology* St. Louis, C.V. Mosby Co., 1976.
4. Shapiro Barry A., Harrison R.A., Walton J.R.: *Clinical Application of Blood Gases*, ed. 2. Chicago, Yearbook Medical Publishers, 1977.

5. Fishman A.P.: *Pulmonary Diseases and Disorders*. New York, McGraw-Hill Book Co., 1980, vol. 1.
6. Fraser R.G., Pare J.A.P.: *Organ Physiology: Structure and Function of the Lung*. Philadelphia, W.B. Saunders Co. 1977.
7. Block J.A.: Low flow oxygen therapy: Treatment of the ambulant outpatient. *Am. Rev. Respir. Dis.* 110:71, 1974.
8. Recommendations for continuous oxygen therapy in chronic lung disease, Committee on Emphysema, American College of Chest Physicians. *Chest* 64:505, 1973.
9. Cherniack R.M., Cherniack L., Naimark A.: *Respiration in Health and Disease*, ed. Z. Philadelphia, W.B. Saunders Co., 1972.
10. Krop H.D., Block A.J., Cohen E.: Neuropsychologic effects of continuous oxygen therapy in chronic obstructive pulmonary disease. *Chest* 64:317, 1973.
11. Kilburn K.H., Dowell A.R.: Renal function in respiratory failure. *Arch. Intern. Med.* 127:754, 1971.
12. Oxygen administration in the Home, American Thoracic Society of the American Lung Association. *Am. Rev. Respir. Dis.* 115:1, 1977.
13. Petty T.L., Stanford R.E., Neff T.A.: Continuous oxygen therapy in chronic airway obstruction. *Ann. Int. Med.* 75:361, 1971.
14. Fox M.J., Snider G.L.: Respiratory therapy: Current practice in ambulatory patients with chronic airflow obstruction. *J.A.M.A.* 241:937, 1979.
15. Continuous or nocturnal oxygen therapy in hypoxemic chronic obstructive lung disease. *Ann. Intern. Med.* 93:391, 1980.
16. Abraham A.S., Cole R.B., Bishop J.M.: Reversal of pulmonary hypertension by prolonged oxygen administration to patients with chronic bronchitis. *Circ. Res.* 23:147, 1968.
17. Mays E.E.: Oxygen therapy in hypoxic chronic bronchitis. *J. Chronic Dis.* 22:421, 1969.
18. Petty T.L., Finigan M.M.: Clinical evaluation of prolonged ambulatory oxygen therapy in chronic airway obstruction. *Am. J. Med.* 45:242, 1968.
19. Levine B.E., Bigelow D.B., Hamstra R.D., et al.: The role of long-term continuous oxygen administration in patients with chronic airway obstruction with hypoxemia. *Ann. Intern. Med.* 66:639, 1967.
20. Gessner D.M.: New developments in oxygen-therapy equipment for home use. *Respir. Ther.*, March 1978.
21. *Medical World News*, July 6, 1981, p. 78.
22. Heimlich H.J.: Respiratory rehabilitation with transtracheal oxygen system. Read before The American Broncho-Esophagological Association Meeting, Palm Beach, Fla., May 4, 1982.
23. Delivering oxygen transtracheally may be a boon for COPD patients. *J.A.M.A.* 248:153, 1982.

9 / Nutrition

DONALD G. BURNS, D.O.

AS IN ALL ASPECTS of pulmonary rehabilitation, nutritional therapy will bolster the patient's resistance against further damage by the disease. Nutritional support will also allow the patient to live with the disease process with a better quality of life.

Poor nutrition occurs quite commonly today in the geriatric population.[1] A rather high percentage of pulmonary rehabilitation patients come from this age group. Malnourishment is often assumed to occur largely in underdeveloped countries where food may not be available, when in actuality malnourishment is often present in individuals who have access to an abundance of food. In the older age group, multiple causes for malnutrition exist. Among these are depression and its resultant anorexia, senility with inability to eat, poor dentition with difficult chewing, and the buying of "junk food" with empty calories, as well as economic factors[1] (see Table 9–1). An optimum rehabilitation program, therefore, must address all these problems and contributing factors.

Metabolic Changes

Chronic obstructive lung disease (COLD) causes several metabolic changes that need to be considered in the rehabilitation plan for the patient. Numerous studies have demonstrated that with increasing severity of COLD, weight progressively decreases.[2] Infection is also a common fac-

TABLE 9–1.—CAUSES OF MALNUTRITION

1. Malabsorption
2. Anorexia caused by the following:
   a. Depression
   b. Drug-induced
   c. Senility
3. Inability to eat because of dyspnea
4. Poor dentition
5. Economic factors
6. Esophageal pathology
7. Ignorance regarding nutritional requirements
8. Catabolism secondary to disease process

135

tor in severe chronic obstructive pulmonary disease and in fact is the most frequent cause of respiratory failure in patients with this disease process.[2]

A vicious cycle may develop with the patient suffering from pulmonary infection and weight loss in that he will suffer progressive malaise, thereby causing increasing anorexia, which will in turn decrease his food intake and contribute to further calorie and protein deficit.

When both weight loss and infection are present concomitantly, protein calorie malnutrition is often present. This protein calorie deficit, if severe, will cause loss of lean body mass with deleterious effects on respiratory muscles as well as on the muscles of locomotion. This may limit the ability to be physically active as well as predispose the individual to respiratory failure. This limitation in physical activity will promote further catabolic activity or inhibit anabolic activity.

Weight loss is secondary to loss of body fat as well as (in severe malnutrition) to protein and lean body mass depletion.[2] The cause of the caloric deficit resulting in weight loss is probably multifactorial. Many times, the patient is depressed and anorexic. Eating may in itself interfere with the breathing process in the severely dyspneic patient. Recent studies have suggested that the patient's total energy requirement is increased as a result of the overall disease process.[2] All these factors may contribute to a gradual weight loss and protein deficit in the patient with COLD.

The disease process may also change the mineral and vitamin requirements. In the hypoxemic patient with increased erythropoietin and erythrocyte production, requirements for iron may be increased. Increased loss of blood through the gastrointestinal (GI) tract is more common in the COLD patient. This may increase iron requirements. Due to the effect of protein malnutrition on the intestinal mucosa, the absorption of vitamins and minerals may also be adversely affected, causing increased requirements for these micronutrients.

In a recent study by Hunter and colleagues[2] it was concluded that in a group of COLD patients with greater than 10% weight loss, the overall nutrient intake exceeded the 1974 Recommended Dietary Allowances of the National Academy of Sciences, National Research Council.[3] This would indicate that this group of patients may have increased requirements for nutrients, including certain vitamins and minerals.

Physiology

The caloric requirement is related to the patient's oxygen requirements as determined by oxygen consumption. A healthy individual requires approximately 3.5 dl of oxygen per kg of body weight per minute at basal conditions. Utilization of 1 L of oxygen releases approximately 5 kcal of heat; therefore, multiplication of the liters of oxygen consumed per day by five will approximate the daily caloric basal requirement. Most individuals will require approximately 30% more oxygen than basal requirements. The following example is that of a 70-kg individual:

$$70 \text{ kg} \times 3.5 \text{ dl/minute} = 245 \text{ dl/min}$$
$$245 \text{ dl} \times 1440 \text{ min/24 hours} = 352.8 \text{ L } 02/24 \text{ hours}$$
$$352.8 \text{ L} \times 5 = 1{,}764 \text{ kcal/24 hours basal}$$
$$1{,}764 \text{ kcal} \times 30\% = 529.2 \text{ kcal}$$
$$1{,}764 \text{ kcal} + 529.2 = 2{,}293 \text{ kcal/24 hours}$$

It has been determined that a deficit of approximately 3,500 calories will result in a 1-lb weight loss. In the example, it can be calculated that a 10% deficit in caloric intake could result in a 24-lb weight loss per year. The same result would be noted with an increase in caloric requirement of 10% without an increase in caloric intake or as follows:

$$2{,}293 \times 10\% = 229.3 \text{ kcal deficit/day}$$
$$229.3 \times 365 \text{ days} = 836{,} 945 \text{ kcal/year deficit}$$
$$836{,} 945 \div 3{,}500 = 23.9 \text{ lb}$$

Pulmonary patients may have problems of increased work of respiration because of increased CO_2 production. Because of abnormal pulmonary mechanics, oxygen consumption may be increased with resultant increased caloric requirements. With increased dead space due to COLD, much of the increased work of respiration would be expended in ventilating this dead space and therefore wasted. This is illustrated by the following example:

Minute ventilation = dead space ventilation + alveolar ventilation
V_D/V_T = 0.3 (normal); therefore,
6 L/min ventilation = 1.8 L dead space + 4.2 alveolar ventilation
V_D/V_T = 0.5 (increased); therefore,
6 L/min ventilation = 3 L dead space + 3 L alveolar ventilation
If the ventilation is increased to 8 L/min:
V_D/V_T = 0.3
8 L = 2.4 L dead space + 5.6 alveolar ventilation
V_D/V_T = 0.5
8 L = 4 L dead space + 4 L alveolar ventilation

It can therefore be calculated that with a V_D/V_T of 0.3, the alveolar ventilation will increase by 1.4 L, whereas the same increase in minute ventilation in the patient with a V_D/V_T of 0.5 will increase the alveolar ventilation by 1 L. This illustrates the inefficiency caused by increased dead space. The decreased efficiency thereby increases work or respiration and the increased tendency toward respiratory failure.

Production of CO_2 is related to metabolism as indicated in the respiratory exchange ratio. When carbohydrate is being metabolized, the oxygen consumed and the CO_2 produced will be equal and the ratio will be 1.0.[5]

$$\text{Glucose} + 6 \text{ O}_2 \rightarrow 6 \text{ CO}_2 + 6 \text{ H}_2\text{O}$$
$$(RQ = 6/6 \text{ or } 1.0)$$

If fat is the fuel being metabolized, the CO_2 produced will be less than the oxygen consumed, and the ratio will, therefore, be less than 1. The ratio with fat would be approximately 0.7.[4]

$$\text{Palmitic acid} + 23 \text{ O}_2 \rightarrow 16 \text{ CO}_2 + 16 \text{ H}_2$$
$$(RQ = 16/23 \text{ or about } 0.7).$$

In a mixed-type diet, the ratio is approximately 0.8. During lipogenesis, the ratio may be greater than 1.[4]

When the supply of oxygen is not sufficient at the cellular level to oxidize fats and glycogen at a sufficiently high rate, lactic acid is produced from the anaerobic metabolism of glycogen. This is expressed in the following equation:

$$\text{Glucose} \rightarrow 2 \text{ La}^- + \text{H}^+$$

The hydrogen ions then react with bicarbonate to form carbonic acid and thus CO_2 as shown below:

$$\text{H}^+ + \text{HCO}_3 \rightarrow \text{CO}_2 + \text{H}_2\text{O}$$

The reaction then causes the bicarbonate level to fall and the CO_2 output to increase.

Any situation in which CO_2 output increases will lead to an increase in ventilation. Included are situations such as a recent heavy meal (which increases CO_2 production because of inhibition of fat metabolism) and any condition tending to impair aerobic metabolism, such as hypoxemia, poor physical fitness, and a poor cardiac response to exercise. In contrast, a reduction in ventilation for a given oxygen consumption accompanies physical training because of decreased CO_2 output, secondary to a lower lactate production.

It has been recognized recently that this difference in CO_2 production with the different nutrients may be very important in the critically ill patient on parenteral nutrition. The high glucose load may adversely effect pH and Pa_{CO_2} if the patient's ventilation is fixed, such as the patient on controlled ventilation.[5]

In the example of our 70-kg reference man with a V_D/V_T ratio of 0.5, it can be seen that by changing the diet from high carbohydrate intake to a mixed-type diet, the amount of ventilation can be decreased by a significant amount, thereby decreasing respiratory work. As noted below, the ventilation required to maintain the arterial CO_2 at 40 torr is 20% less with a mixed diet than with a carbohydrate diet:

$$70 \text{ kg} \times 3.5 = 245 \text{ dl } O_2/\text{min}$$

$$245 \text{ dl } O_2 \times 1 = 245 \text{ dl } CO_2/\text{min on carbohydrate diet}$$

$$\text{Alveolar ventilation} = \frac{CO_2 \text{ production} \times 0.863}{\text{arterial } CO_2}$$

$$V_A = \frac{245 \times 0.863}{40} = 5.2 \text{ L/min}$$

$$\text{Minute ventilation} = \frac{5.2}{0.5} = 10.4 \text{ L/min}$$

$$245 \text{ dl } O_2 \times 0.8 = 196 \text{ dl } CO_2/\text{min on a mixed diet}$$

$$V_A = \frac{196 \times 0.863}{40} = 4.2 \text{ L/min}$$

$$\text{Minute ventilation} = \frac{4.2}{0.5} = 8.4 \text{ L/min}$$

$$10.4 - 8.4 = 2.0$$

$$\frac{2.0}{10.4} = 19\% \text{ less ventilation with mixed diet}$$

When the problems of increased CO_2 production and increased dead space in the COLD patient are compounded, one can see that the increased ventilation required over that of an individual with normal lungs is considerable. The previous example assumes maintenance of the arterial CO_2 at a constant level. If the patient's respiratory muscles fatigue at this level of ventilation, then respiratory failure may occur.

Protein depletion of the *marasmic* skeletal muscle type is the most common type of protein depletion in the COLD patient. In this situation, skeletal muscle atrophy occurs. This may cause weakness of the respiratory muscles, predisposing the patient to inspiratory muscle fatigue. Inspiratory muscle fatigue then predisposes the patient to respiratory failure and all of its physiologic consequences.

If severe protein depletion occurs, visceral protein deficiency may be present of the *kwashiorkor* (visceral protein depletion) type. The patient in this situation will be especially susceptible to infection. If the patient has an isolated kwashiorkor protein malnutrition, at first glance he may appear relatively healthy. He may actually be obese; however, there is a thin malnourished body beneath the obvious obesity. Occasionally this same type of situation can occur with a marasmic type of protein malnutrition.

Micronutrient deficiency occurs in many geriatric patients, including those with COLD.[1] Deficiencies of the micronutrients may predispose an individual to numerous problems including infection, muscle fatigue, and problems in other organ systems (Table 9–2).

Nutritional Assessment

As part of a comprehensive rehabilitation program for the pulmonary patient, it is important to have an accurate and complete data base. From this data base, a rational and effective program for the individual patient can be developed. This assessment should be based on physiologic principles and individualized as much as possible. A comprehensive history regarding nutrition and complete physical examination may allow deletion of much of the laboratory examination in individual patients. With the high cost of many laboratory studies, this is an important consideration; however, one must not be "penny wise and pound foolish" in this regard. Skipping necessary tests may in the end not only cost more dollars, but be very dangerous for the patient.

The nutritional assessment will, in a relatively simple manner, allow the collection of necessary data to develop an optimal nutritional program. In evaluation of the nutritional status, four areas need to be examined:

ENERGY STORES.—Energy stores are best measured by anthropometric means. The relationship of the patient's actual weight to ideal weight reflects overall energy stores. Triceps skin fold measurements give an indication of energy stores in fat tissue. This test is quite crude and must be cautiously interpreted.

SOMATIC MUSCLE STORES.—These are measured by 24-hour urinary creatinine excretion. From this measurement, a creatinine/height index can be calculated. This is usually expressed as a percent of standard that is obtained from available tables.

VISCERAL PROTEIN STORES.—These are measured by serum albumin. Severe malnutrition is indicated by a serum albumin of less than 3.0 gm/dl. Transferrin levels may also be helpful. The lower limits of normal are 170 mg/dl.

TABLE 9–2.—TYPES OF MALNUTRITION

---

1. Caloric deficit
2. Protein deficiency
   a. Visceral (kwashiorkor)
   b. Muscle (marasmic)
3. Micronutrient deficiency
   a. Vitamin
   b. Mineral
4. Combined

HOST DEFENSE MECHANISM.—Evidence of anergy as indicated by failure to respond to a battery of skin tests, as well as a total lymphocyte count of less than 1,500, points to kwashiorkor type of malnutrition or visceral protein depletion.

Protein starvation is very common in the chronic-diseased patient. In hospitalized general medical patients, 44% have protein-energy malnutrition.[6] The organs most affected are those with rapid protein turnover rates. These include the hematopoietic system, the GI system, and the skin. A "flaky-paint" type of dermatitis is common in patients with protein deficiency. The effect on the GI system includes mucosal cell defects, which may result in malabsorption of certain macronutrients as well as micronutrients (vitamins and minerals). This causes a vicious cycle with increasing malnutrition. The cell-mediated immune responses are also profoundly affected; therefore, skin tests are useful in evaluation. IgA levels may also be reduced. Stem-cell proliferation is affected and causes an impaired ability to mount neutrophil responses to infection.

The method by which a nutritional assessment is performed may vary. At the present time, the following method is practical and adequate:

Initial Assessment

1. *History.*—Detailed history regarding dietary habits, past weight, change in weight.

2. *Physical Examination.*—General appearance, skin.

3. *Anthropometric.*—Height, weight, triceps skin fold measurement, mid arm muscle circumference.

4. *Laboratory.*—24-hour urinary creatinine, serum albumin, transferrin, total lymphocyte count.

5. *Skin Tests.*—Candida, mumps, trichophyton, streptokinase, purified protein derivative.

6. *Miscellaneous (if available).*—Oxygen consumption, CO_2 production, respiratory exchange ratio.

After the initial studies are done, it is important that they be repeated periodically after the nutritional program is instituted so the program's effect can be monitored. The frequency with which the studies should be repeated will depend largely on the individual patient. If the patient does not appear to be responding to therapy, it may be necessary to monitor the studies more frequently; however, in the outpatient on a rehabilitation program, every 6 to 8 weeks is generally sufficient.

Nutritional Therapy

The nutritional management of the pulmonary patient must be individualized. This individualization must take into account not only the physiologic needs of the patient, but also his likes and dislikes. In the rehabilitation patient, the nutrients will usually be eaten, unlike the critically ill patient where the nutrients may have to be administered by either total parenteral nutrition or by enteric feeding tubes. Preferably, the patient will eat a normal type of diet; however, often it will be necessary to supplement the diet with modules of nutrients such as protein, fat, or carbohydrate. Supplementary use of the micronutrients are also often desirable.

In the pulmonary patient's diet prescription, there are several things that need to be considered. First, what are the patient's caloric requirements? This may be determined from measurement of the patient's oxygen consumption or, more often, from estimations of oxygen consumption. If the individual has a basal oxygen consumption of 3.5 dl/kg and weighs 70 kg, it can be calculated that the basal oxygen consumption is 245 dl/min. Multiplying this by the 1,440 min in 24 hours, the daily oxygen consumption would, therefore, be approximately 353 L.

Because utilization of 1 L of oxygen will produce approximately 5 kcal, one may multiply 353 L by five to obtain an approximate basal caloric requirement of 1,765 kcal. Add approximately 30% of this basal requirement for minimal activity above basal levels, and the caloric requirements are approximately 2,300 calories per day.

The pulmonary patient's weight should be maintained as close to ideal as possible. As a rule of thumb, this may be calculated by subtracting 60 from the patient's height in inches. This figure is then multiplied by five and added to 100 for females and 110 for males.

If the patient's weight is not near ideal, it may then be desirable to calculate either a decrease or an increase in calories to help bring the weight to a desired level. Normally, 3,500 calories equals 1 lb of fat; therefore, one may multiply the number of pounds the patient needs to gain or lose by 3,500 to obtain the total caloric change needed. This may then be divided by the number of days over which the weight change should occur and either add or subtract from the basal caloric need.

The pulmonary patient's diet should be constructed so as to keep CO_2 production to a minimum. This means trying to keep the respiratory exchange ratio as low as practical. Since eating carbohydrates will create six molecules of CO_2 for every six molecules of oxygen utilized, it can be seen that carbohydrates should be kept to a minimum. Fat metabolism, on the other hand, produces only 70% as much CO_2 as oxygen consumed and would be desirable from this standpoint. Cardiovascular and other considerations, however, may limit this desirability.

Approximately 40% to 45% of calories in the normal American diet are derived from fat and essentially the same percentage from carbohydrates. It can therefore be seen that the use of fats for energy is as important as the use of carbohydrates. An average of 30% to 50% of the carbohydrates ingested with each meal is converted to triglycerides, stored, and later utilized as energy. Therefore, a high percentage of the energy utilized directly by the cells might be supplied by triglycerides.

The fats in the diet should be of the unsaturated rather than the saturated type when possible. This would indicate the eating of vegetable fats as well as putting emphasis in the diet on fish and poultry, rather than on beef and pork.

After consideration of the total caloric requirements and the type of foodstuffs that are desired, protein requirements should then be calculated. If no evidence of protein depletion is seen in the patient, then approximately 0.8 gm/kg body weight should be adequate. If protein depletion is present, either of the marasmic or kwashiorkor type, then it will be necessary to do a nitrogen balance study and give enough protein to bring the patient into positive balance. This would entail doing 24-hour urinary urea nitrogen studies and calculating the protein loss per 24 hours. An approximate 100% increase in this amount should then be given to allow gradual improvement in the protein depletion.

Nitrogen balance compares the amount of dietary nitrogen taken in minus the nitrogen excreted. The nitrogen intake is simply the amount of protein ingested per day divided by 6.25 (number taken in = grams protein/6.25). The nitrogen loss may be estimated by 24-hour measurement of urinary urea nitrogen (UUN). A factor of 2 gm/day is then added to the UUN to account for nonurea-nitrogen losses such as creatinine, ammonia, urea acids, etc. To this figure is added an additional 2 gm for fecal and skin losses. The nitrogen balance is then calculated by subtracting the nitrogen output from the nitrogen taken in. If the patient's blood urea nitrogen (BUN) changes in the 24 hours during collection, this must be taken into account and calculated as gram change in 24 hours and added to the gram-nitrogen output.[7]

For example, a 70-kg man with a BUN change of 10 mg/dl in a 24-hour period, 24 hours UUN 8 gm, protein intake of 100 gm/day would have the following calculated nitrogen balance:

$$N_{in} = 100 \text{ gm}/6.25 = 16 \text{ gm N}$$
$$N_{out} = 8 \text{ gm UUN} + (10 \text{ mg/dl} \times 0.60 \ (70 \text{ kg}) \times 0.01) + 4$$
$$N_{out} = 8 + 4.2 + 4 = 16.2$$
$$N_{bal} = 16 - 16.2 = -0.2$$

Micronutrients must also be given consideration in the nutritional plan. As noted, micronutrient absorption may be affected by the protein deficiencies' effect on the intestinal mucosa. The changing American diet, with more emphasis on fast foods and foods processed by chemical means, certainly affects the availability and metabolism of micronutrients. One example is that of calcium. In the past 25 years, the intake of phosphorus has greatly increased in relation to calcium in the diet. A high percentage of the geriatric population is in negative calcium balance. This population is the population in which the pulmonary patients are most prevalent. Vitamin deficiency may also be present in this population of patients.[1]

Supplementation of the diet with vitamins and minerals is generally believed to be useful in the majority of COLD patients. Multiple B vitamins with vitamin C is probably the most useful combination. The dosage of vitamins and minerals should usually be approximately the recommended daily allowance. No real advantage has been documented for megadoses. Calcium in a dosage of 0.5 to 1.0 gm daily is also recommended. This is usually given in either the carbonate or gluconate form.

Summary

Rehabilitation of the pulmonary patient requires a multifaceted approach. The nutritional status of the patient is important to the ultimate success of the rehabilitation plan. The success of a nutritional program in the overall rehabilitation of the patient with COLD depends on its individualization to the particular needs of the patient. The etiologic factors for malnutrition in the pulmonary patient are physiologic, economic, educational, dental, and mental; and the treatment program must vary to reach the goal of optimum rehabilitation.

Total caloric requirements must be determined and met in the patient. The protein requirements should then be determined and a plan for meeting these undertaken. The micronutrients are also quite important to the overall well-being of the pulmonary patient.

Much has been written regarding the nutritional management of the critically ill pulmonary patient. The nutritional management of the patient in that situation may truly determine life or death. The outcome in the chronically ill may be less dramatic, but is, nevertheless, of the same magnitude. The quality of life is very likely the most evident benefit of an optimum nutritional program.

References

1. Kohrs M.B., O'Neal R., Preston A., et al.: Nutritional status of elderly residents of Missouri. *Am. J. Clin. Nutr.* 31:2186, 1978.
2. Hunter A.M., Carey M.A., Larsh H.W.: The nutritional status of patients with chronic obstructive pulmonary disease. *Am. Rev. Respir. Dis.* 124:376, 1981.
3. Munro H.N.: Nutritional requirements in health. *Crit. Care Med.* 8:2, 1979.
4. Guyton A.C.: *Textbook of Medical Physiology*, ed. 4. Philadelphia, W.B. Saunders Co., 1971.

5. Askanazi J., Rosenbaum S., Hyman A., et al.: Effects of total parenteral nutrition on gas exchange and breathing patterns. *Crit. Care Med.* 7:125, 1979.
6. Wright R.A.: Nutritional assessment. *J.A.M.A.* 244:559, 1980.
7. Bennoti P., Blackburn G.L.: Protein and caloric or macronutrient metabolic management of the critically ill patient. *Crit. Care Med.* 7:520, 1979.

10 / Psychosocial Factors in Pulmonary Rehabilitation*

JACK K. PLUMMER, Ph.D.

DUE TO THE HIGH INCIDENCE of pulmonary disease, easier access to health and social programs, effective diagnostic and treatment techniques affecting morbidity and mortality, and the (as yet unspecified) effects of exposure to environmental pollutants, respiratory health problems and pulmonary disability have increased dramatically. In addition to the tremendous medical problems associated with pulmonary disease, the psychosocial impact on the patient and family is severe, thus affecting the "quality of life." This has created a need for sophisticated, comprehensive, multidisciplinary rehabilitation approaches. Such approaches are based on scientific knowledge and the application of a variety of treatment techniques by a team of professionals working in concert with the patient and family. An indispensable portion of this "rehabilitation philosophy" rests upon the complete understanding of the psychosocial elements involved in adaptation to chronic respiratory insufficiency.

As an historic example of early efforts in this direction, asthma and allergic reactions have been heavily researched and described in the literature for 30 years. In 1953, Leigh[1] critically analyzed the role of psychological factors in asthma, stressing the importance of moving beyond mere descriptive discourse to more scientific, longitudinal analysis. A year later, Dunbar[2] provided a comprehensive review of the literature from 1910 to 1953 pertaining to the relationships between emotions and respiratory physiology. In a review of the clinical and experimental literature, Freeman and associates[3] focused on respiratory allergies, asthmatic rhinitis, and hayfever, with special emphasis on methodological issues. The authors properly pointed out that psychological variables had been viewed as etiologic factors or as concomitants in these disorders for many years. Several categories of approaches to attendant issues were highlighted, and many assumptions, methodologies, and generalizations were questioned.

---

*Expanded from a presentation at the American Association of Respiratory Therapy Annual Convention, New Orleans, November 2, 1982.

Other writings have assigned psychological variables to the etiology of either allergies in general or to asthma or bronchitis in particular. Psychosis, schizophrenia, psychosomatic disorders, narcotics addiction, and alcoholism have appeared in the literature, with various psychoanalytic, psychosomatic, and other psychological theories associated with each physiologic and behavioral connection. One study viewed asthma as a learned response developed initially through conditioning and maintained through anxiety reduction as reinforcement.[4] Psychogenic hypotheses of specific vulnerability have been of interest in that individuals are posited to have certain predispositions established by heredity and life experience that emerge in psychosomatic syndromes as a result of psychological stress. Likewise, some research has been carried out to identify subgroups with different psychological makeups within an allergic population. Although these are certainly promising approaches, with few exceptions[5, 6] little evidence exists to identify psychological differences accompanying various illnesses. The most that can be said based on studies up to 20 years ago is that "the allergic population is far from homogeneous psychologically, and the role of psychological variables varies in subgroups of patients with allergic symptoms."[3] Therefore, whether psychosocial factors are etiologic ingredients or precipitants, they have played a prominent role in the treatment of asthma and allergic reactions, far above that derived from a basic immunologic model.

More recently, Dirks and others[7-26] have constituted a research group in Colorado with a prolific series of studies of personality/situational variables in asthma, especially panic-fear behavior constellations. These researchers have been particularly interested in the medical intractability of asthma and its relationship to the demand for and utilization of medical services, request for medication, length of hospitalization, and recidivism rates. They refer to "psychomaintenance," the perpetuation of chronic illness, or the "failure" of medical treatment because of psychological, as opposed to strictly physical, causes. Other studies have concentrated on anxiety and depression[27] and coping styles.[26] Much writing has also appeared in the area of adolescents,[28] children,[29, 30] and their families.[31-34] To present further analysis of these areas would require additional chapters.

One noteworthy theoretic treatment of bronchial asthma has been offered by Groen,[35] who discusses this respiratory disorder as a paradigm of theory in psychosomatic medicine. Response predisposition developed through an interaction of heredity and environment, including overprotection by a domineering parent, plays a major role. The resultant behavioral inhibition then gets played out in physical/physiologic changes in the pulmonary system, namely, obstruction of the large airways. By these mechanisms, the author explains bronchial hyperreactivity and secondary development of allergies.

Less prominent than asthma, but nonetheless important in the field, is discourse concerning chronic bronchitis. For example, Rutter[36-38] discusses this disorder within the broader context of the development of chronic illness along with its many psychological concomitants. He has demonstrated differences between bronchitic patients and nonbronchitic controls in both psychiatric disturbance and "neurotic" personality traits.

No less important, but also not appearing in the pulmonary literature as often as a specific disease entity, is lung cancer. This is interesting, because lung cancer accounted for more than 25% of all cancer deaths in 1982, amounting to 111,000 people (6,000 more than the previous year). The death rate from lung cancer is rising spectacularly in comparison with the death rates of other cancers such as colorectal, breast, and uterine types.[39] Furthermore, lung cancer is extremely fatal, with only 9% to 10% of those diagnosed living 5 years or more. Reportedly, cigarette smoking increases the risk of lung cancer tenfold, and 75% of this cancer can be prevented by not smoking.[39, 40] Hence, lung cancer is quite preventable when compared with other cancer types, and there are many implications for psychosocial factors, not only for prevention, but also for treatment. In one study, intervention successfully ameliorated psychosocial problems of cancer patients, such as decreasing anxiety, hostility, and depression and facilitating a more realistic outlook on life and a more constructive lifestyle. Patients with lung cancer required the most service, and the authors state that it is important to view cancer as a group of different diseases with differing impact on the person, thus requiring a different type of adaptation and intervention.[41] Usually, however, psychosocial aspects of cancer are not dealt with according to the site,[42-45] and the impact on the family, as well as the patient, is not often systematically addressed. An exception is a model developed by Giacquinta[46] based on an analysis of 100 families facing cancer. The author includes stages of impact, functional disruption, a search for meaning, informing others, engaging emotions, reorganization, and framing memories.

Unfortunately, however, with the exception of asthma, relatively little attention has been devoted in practice or in the literature to psychosocial aspects of pulmonary rehabilitation. For example, a major symposium over 10 years ago in rehabilitation of the "pulmonary cripple" (an opprobrious term that has since been abandoned, gave short shrift to psychosocial considerations in both inpatient[47] and outpatient programs[48] as well as private practice.[49] Some mention was made of patient and family education and of personality characteristics of the emphysema patient in a presentation on vocational rehabilitation.[50] Writings in other disciplines have in the past reflected the same lack of attention in nursing,[51] physical therapy,[52] and respiratory therapy.[53] On the other hand, articles in occupational therapy, a field with a traditionally broader scope, discussed depression and anxiety due to the "double insult" of disease and aging. Acceptance of disability, self-assurance, diversion, objectivity, patient and family education, activities of daily living, self-responsibility, and a healthful balance among work, leisure, and rest were worthy inclusions.[54, 55] Another exception written by a physician (published 15 years ago) discussed "mental" aspects of chronic obstructive lung disease (COLD), mostly depression, but importantly pointed out the impact of respiratory disease of lifestyle.[56]

One of the first articles highlighting nonmedical aspects of pulmonary rehabilitation was by Fishman and Petty,[57] and others appeared by Dudley, Wermuth and Hague[58] and Backus and Dudley,[59] authors who have continued to be quite active in promoting a comprehensive approach entailing not only important physical, physiologic and medical aspects, but psychosocial ones as well.[60-65] For example, the reciprocal relationships between emotional states and pulmonary physiology create a precarious balance for respiratory patients, causing them to live in an emotional "straightjacket."[58] This causes severe coping problems not only for the patients and families, but also for the professionals who work with them.

An earlier article was written by two psychologists and a physician about the neuropsychologic effects of continuous oxygen therapy in COLD.[66] Later, a similar article published in the same journal applied to a sample of 19 older men with a mean age of 71.[67] This preliminary, intriguing research stimulated new concepts in pulmonary rehabilitation, because it highlighted the important role of respiratory therapy in possibly improving cognitive functioning.

More recently, at the 22nd Aspen Lung Conference in 1979, Grant and others[68] described some observations of neuropsychologic states with a much larger sample of hypoxemic COLD patients as part of the Nocturnal Oxygen Therapy Trial. It is interesting to note, in keeping with an earlier point, that this conference summary[69] did not even touch on psychosocial factors, even in a section on the response of the individual to the disease. Instead, the focus was on *technical* aspects of breathlessness, a symptom that is most terrifying to the patient and family and very anxiety-producing in caregivers. A section on interventions gave only passing mention to emotional disturbances and reduction in the quality of life. Likewise, a major monograph of the proceedings of the conference on the scientific basis of in-hospital respiratory therapy held in Atlanta in 1979 barely alludes to comprehensive care (in one article), but this does not entail psychosocial applications.[53]

It is hoped that the "state of the art" described in these publications 3 years ago has somehow become more all-inclusive and thus humanistic, but skepticism remains for such fulfillment in the near future. Significant departures from a narrow, medical view have been a thought-provoking address by Vanderpool[70] on "Health Care for the Whole Person" in which he stresses the need for continuously examining ethical issues in the training of professionals and patient treatment and a discussion on "Pulmonary Rehabilitation" by Scoggins and Simpson,[71] both delivered at the 1982 American Association for Respiratory Therapy Annual Convention. These efforts are more in keeping with the definition adopted by the Committee on Pulmonary Rehabilitation of the American College of Chest Physicians at its annual meeting in 1974, referred to in the opening pages of this book.

An impressive illustration of a holistic conceptualization is a current monograph edited by Hodgkin,[72] resulting from an extensive review of pulmonary medicine and related areas by a task force formulated by the Human Interaction Research Institute and funded by a grant from the National Science Foundation. Therapeutic modalities required for the comprehensive care of patients with COLD include patient and family education, adequate fluid intake, proper nutrition, and avoidance of infections and inhaled irritants (such as through smoking). Also considered in the discussion are use of medications, respiratory therapy, environmental stress, lifestyle, and goal-setting, and patient motivation and other psychological states.

Hodgkin[72] states, "The benefits that can be demonstrated if the physician uses comprehensive and systematic respiratory care include a decrease in the frequency and duration of hospital admissions; socioeconomic gains from reduced hospitalizations; a reduction in anxiety, depression, and somatic concern; the return of some patients to positions of employment; and the establishment of a better quality of life. Persistence by physicians, allied health workers and families is essential to support the patient in a continued systematic program of treatment. . ." Thus, the emphasis in this chapter will be on a comprehensive, multidisciplinary approach involving dietetics, medicine, nursing, psychology, vocational rehabilitation, and occupational, physical, recreational, and respiratory therapies. An excellent example within an urban hospital setting is offered by Dr. Albert A. Haas and his associates, derived from the results of two Rehabilitation Services Administration-funded developmental rehabilitation programs.[73] From their study of severely disabled COLD patients who were provided comprehensive pulmonary rehabilitation services over a 5-year period, the investigators found that 25% of the sample was able to return to full, gainful employment, whereas only 3% of the control group was able to do so. According to the authors of this monograph, several measures need to be taken if the lives of COLD patients are to improve significantly. These changes need to be reflected not only in the attitudes of allied health professionals, but also in the policies at local, regional, and national levels.

Let us turn now to some discussion of a "quality of life" model that is useful in stressing the desired comprehensive nature of pulmonary rehabilitation. In 1974, sociologist Anselm Strauss pointed out that despite the debilitating, degenerative, and eventually fatal aspects of chronic disease, medical care continues to focus on symptomatic relief and dealing with acute phases of illness. Strauss[74] stated that patients, in contrast, are more often concerned with preserving or maintaining quality of life than with the nature of their disease.

Agle and Baum[75] correctly argue that being cognizant of psychosocial aspects of pulmonary care and engaging in psychological intervention does not replace damaged lung tissue. Nevertheless, beyond the goal of prolongation of life is the goal so important to the patient and family, that of daily function and reasonable comfort, in effect, "the quality of life."

The quality of life is specifically addressed in three 1982 articles. Using the results of a survey of 500 men and 500 women, encompassing 6,500 activities and experiences, Flanagan[76] ultimately factored out 15 components that were considered most significant by the subjects (Table 10–1).

Based on these results, he proposed that a new set of dimensions be applied to disabled persons, dimensions based on their needs and changes that can be made to produce the greatest improvement in the quality of life.

Discussing philosophic considerations in a companion article, Kottke[77] focuses on meaningful interpersonal relationships and personal participation yielding a sense of self-fulfillment. From a social work perspective, Caputi[78] points out that the underlying issue is how professionals in health care can maintain humanistic aspects of healing while providing the benefits of a highly developed medical technology. With a strong patient/family rights flavor, Caputi[78] emphasizes the enhancement of *coping skills*.

In another 1982 article[79] that was included in the collaborative NOTT study mentioned earlier, psychologists and physicians define "quality of life" as encompassing four dimensions: (1) emotional functioning, (2) social-

TABLE 10–1.—COMPONENTS OF THE QUALITY OF LIFE*

MOST IMPORTANT DIMENSIONS	NEEDS LEAST WELL MET	QUALITY OF LIFE FACTORS
1. Health	1. Participation in government	1. Material comforts
2. Children	2. Active recreation	2. Work
3. Understanding oneself	3. Learning and education	3. Health
4. Work	4. Creative expression	4. Active recreation
5. Relationship with spouse	5. Helping others	5. Learning and education

*Adapted from Flanagan J.C.: Measurement of quality of life: Current state of the art. *Arch. Phys. Med. Rehabil.* 63:56-59, 1982.

role functioning, including home management and social and family relationships, (3) activities of daily living, such as self-care skills and mobility, and (4) the ability to engage in enjoyable hobbies and other recreational pastimes.

Data from self-reports and reports from spouses or close relatives of the patient revealed that the life quality of patients with COLD was impaired in almost all respects. Depression, anxiety, social isolation, and decreased leisure-time activities were observed in the majority of the sample when compared with healthy controls. Age, socioeconomic status, and neuropsychological functioning were important moderators or facilitators of coping ability. McSweeny and coworkers[79] developed a heuristic model depicting the interrelation of COLD and variables affecting the quality of life (Fig 10–1).

Similar to an earlier suggestion by Dudley and associates,[61] the McSweeny group[79, 80] proposes integrating psychosocial supports into a multimodal pulmonary rehabilitation program. They believe that psychological interventions that are a routine part of patient and family education and therapy become less obtrusive and thereby more acceptable. Moreover, in a report of a 15-month patient education study prepared for the American Lung Association, Seiler[81] indicated that educational programs elicit positive and apparently significant and long-lasting changes in the COLD patient's psychological well-being.

Louis Post, a former staff psychologist at Gaylord Hospital, Wallingford,

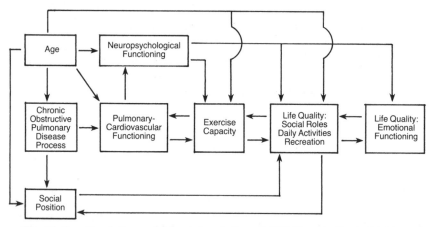

Fig 10–1.—Heuristic model for interrelation of COLD and other variables affecting life quality. (From McSweeny A.J., Grant I., Heaton R.K., et al.: Life quality of patients with chronic obstructive pulmonary disease. *Arch. Intern. Med.* 142:477, 1982; copyright 1982, American Medical Association. Used by permission.)

Conn., and his associate, Claire Collins,[82] a nurse practitioner, discussed an etiology of maladaptive coping in COLD and a model for psychotherapeutic intervention that aims at (1) facilitating acceptance of losses and restructuring life goals, (2) interrupting the cycle of alienation and social withdrawal, and (3) increasing the patient's control over affective arousal and respiratory functioning. The application of individual, family, and couple therapy and specific behavioral techniques are discussed by Post and Collins[82] as being useful in promoting more adaptive coping in the COLD patient.

A Paradigm of Pulmonary Rehabilitation

One of several special-care units within a 121-bed, free-standing complex, Gaylord's unit for the treatment of respiratory insufficiency consists of 23 inpatient beds, a 4-bed cardiopulmonary monitoring unit, and outpatient services including a weekly pulmonary clinic. Gaylord has been strongly committed to a multidisciplinary team approach for 15 years, and disciplines involved in the treatment of respiratory insufficiency include dietary, medicine, nursing, psychology, social work, and occupational, physical, recreational, and respiratory therapies as well as many other medical and rehabilitation specialities.

Psychosocial factors are taken into account even before the patient's admission at Gaylord. The nurse, physician, psychologist, and social worker may collaborate in the admissions process, depending upon an assessment of the preadmission data. For example, in the case of the patient who may have the potential of becoming ventilator-dependent, a conference is held in which the professionals, patient, and family participate in arriving at decisions regarding the possibility of a tracheostomy and future discharge planning.

The Multidisciplinary Team Approach

There are four basic assumptions underlying the multidisciplinary team:

1. A team is a group of professionals engaged in a process of decision making with patients and families, all of whom share a common purpose in meeting together and sharing knowledge from which plans are made and therapeutic decisions are influenced.[83]

2. A team enables each member, including the patient and family, to contribute maximally to treatment through the centralization of decision making, power, and authority and encourages more open feedback of important information.

3. Unless a team member assumes responsibility for defining his or her area of responsibility, authority, and competence to other team members, the team is a myth.[83]

4. It should be recognized and accepted that the solution to a treatment facility's many problems does not lie exclusively in the use of the team, but rather that more effective understanding and treatment of patients can be facilitated through the use of team principles.

Generally, disregarding the aforementioned assumptions can lead to a number of common problems that interfere with effective team functioning, such as nonallegiance to team models; building rigidities and professional imperialism; the pursuit of individual vs. team goals; failure to include the patient and/or family in decision making; bureaucratic demands; and assorted individual, team, patient, family, and organizational idiosyncracies, deficiencies, and incompetencies. A comprehensive, multidisciplinary team approach is the therapeutic model of choice, but this requires much more than lip service or an "in name only" pseudo-team model. The advantages of this approach include (1) reciprocal stimulation by the team members, (2) convening of a pool of resources and accumulation of skills, (3) an increase in the probability of developing and using insight, (4) cancellation of many potential errors, (5) correction of "blind spots" and other sources of bias, and (6) development of a sense of security and a useful increase of risk taking.

At Gaylord, the various team members participate in patient/family education. Topics include instruction in the following:

1. anatomy and physiology
2. diaphragmatic breathing
3. relaxation training
4. pharmacologic management
5. assistive breathing devices
6. the intricacies of blood gases
7. postural drainage
8. nutrition and diet
9. stretching and posture
10. work simplification
11. energy conservation
12. pacing
13. activities of daily living
14. use of leisure time
15. sexuality
16. issues concerning Social Security benefits and third-party payment
17. other assorted subjects designed to enhance coping strategies

A pulmonary education program is held every Wednesday evening on the pulmonary unit. The first half of the meeting consists of a presentation by staff, and the second part consists of discussion of problems and issues surrounding pulmonary disability and rehabilitation. Patients and families are invited, and staff and other speakers participate.

Self-Help Groups

Self-help and other mutual support groups have been impressive additions to other types of intervention with a variety of ailments, illnesses, diseases, and conditions. Self-help groups have been defined as "voluntary small group structures for mutual aid in the accomplishment of a specific purpose. They are usually formed by peers who have come together for mutual assistance and satisfying a common need, overcoming a common handicap or life-disrupting problem, in bringing about desired social and/or personal change."[84] It has been estimated that such mutual-aid groups total about 500,000, involving more than 15,000,000 people.[85] In 1981, a special survey on selected hospital topics documented that 48.3% of the nation's hospitals reported one or more active self-help groups, and a follow-up questionnaire revealed that the sample of hospitals listed an average of 5.65 self-help support groups per hospital. Cancer support groups ranked the highest and stroke clubs the lowest, with support groups associated with respiratory care in the middle. Respondents identified the primary benefit to the hospital as improved public relations and community visibility. The benefits for staff fell into three categories: increased ability to deliver quality care, more satisfying relationships with patients, and increased job satisfaction. The patients indicated that they benefitted from emotional support, decreased anxiety, better acceptance of the disease, and more effective coping. Improved continuity of care, greater availability of support groups, and a greater likelihood of a needed referral were also included.[86]

There is literally no problem group that has not been touched in some way by this type of assistance, namely those associated with alcoholism, schizophrenia, learning disabilities, heart disease, diabetes, muscular dystrophy, mental retardation, mental illness, obesity, cerebral palsy, and Guillain-Barré syndrome as well as child-abusing parents, the aged, gamblers, people with gay/lesbian sexual preferences, autistic children, single parents and their children, and smokers. Categorizing all of these groups gives rise to three types: (1) self-care groups for those suffering from physical and mental illness, (at least one group for nearly every major disease), (2) the reform groups for addictive behaviors such as Alcoholics Anonymous, Gamblers Anonymous, and Overeaters Anonymous, and (3) advocacy groups for certain minorities, the elderly, homosexuals, the physically disabled, and so on.[87]

There are several useful sources for obtaining information on self-help groups.[85, 87-90] Also, organizations in an increasing number of states are collecting and disseminating information about local self-help groups and resources, coordinated by the National Self-Help Clearing House (Graduate School and University Center/CUNY, 33 W. 42 St., New York, N.Y. 10036).

Gartner and Riessman,[91] codirectors of the National Self-Help Clearing House, add the following to the description of these groups:

1. Self-help groups always involve face-to-face interactions.

2. Personal participation is extremely important, since bureaucratization is the enemy of the self-help organization.

3. Members agree on and engage in some actions.

4. Typically, the groups start from a condition of powerlessness.

5. The groups fill needs for a reference group, a point of connection and identification with others, a base for activity, and a source of ego reinforcement. The authors further point out that these groups have unique preventive features: they "provide social support to their members through the creation of a caring community, and they increase members' coping skills through the provision of information and the sharing of experiences and solutions to problems."[91]

The enhancement of coping skills is specifically addressed by Durman,[92] focusing on the "need for human interaction, available quickly in crisis, at all hours, for potentially long periods of time, in which the focus is not basic change in the outlook or personality, but in sustaining the ability to cope with a difficult situation."

Based on five factors characteristic of any medical encounter contributing to fear, dread, and apprehension (dependency, loss of control, changed behavioral norms, fear, and concerns about others' responses), DeMocker and Zimpfer[93] describe several contributions of group work in psychosocial intervention. These include the following:

1. providing information

2. broadening perspective

3. providing emotional catharsis

4. providing peer support

5. improving interpersonal communications

6. expanding social role

7. facilitating the practice of self-care

8. providing modeling

9. helping group member to confront reality

An exemplary self-help group is the 6-year-old Gaylord Respiratory Club, cosponsored by the hospital and the American Lung Association of Connecticut. Two staff liaisons (one from Recreation Therapy and one from Psychology) meet regularly with the club's Steering Committee and serve as consultants to the group. This self-help group provides educational programs contributing to self-care and has produced a book called *Around the Clock With COPD*,[94] which is distributed to all inpatients and members of the club. Meetings also provide practical suggestions, opportunities for socializing, focus on economic and social issues, and emotional support to help the participants adapt more effectively through empathy and improved interpersonal communication. Advocacy is also an activity of the group, including lobbying for changes in legislation appropriate to their situations. The Gaylord Division of Psychology facilitated the founding of the Respiratory Club and continues to enhance its contribution to pulmonary rehabilitation.

Death and Dying: Patients' Rights

Another psychosocial aspect involved in pulmonary rehabilitation is the issue of patient rights as they relate to death and dying. This issue is perhaps uncomfortable for professionals and family members alike, but it must be dealt with responsibly. For decades in this society, death has been a taboo topic; consequently, many of us have generally avoided talking about it. Only recently have these barriers begun to come down through the publication of numerous books and articles and a growing recognition in the professional community that those people intimately involved with death often need help in dealing with it. It is very difficult to separate the issue of the patient's right to *die* from the patient's right to *know*. Controversy continues to surround the latter topic in spite of various pertinent publications within treatment facilities and the adoption of patient rights legislation throughout the country. The so-called Patient's Bill of Rights began with efforts by the American Hospital Association in 1972 and was approved by their House of Delegates Feb. 6, 1973. Much support for this concept has appeared in the professional as well as in the public media over the years. However, some empiric support has also been generated. At a New England hospital, for example, over a period of several months, every patient on the Rehabilitation Medicine service received a carbon copy of Admission and Discharge notes based on the Problem Oriented Medical Record.[95] The response on the part of the patients and staff was positive, with few reported problems emanating from this policy. Moreover, the authors conclude that this procedure aids the rehabilitation process by providing for orderly, shared participation and responsibility within the medical care system. A later article made use of similar feedback in promoting patients' rights and effective treatment.[96] More recently, Altman and coworkers[97] observed that freedom of information is not the only issue in gaining access to one's own medical record, but this also involves trust/mistrust, dissatisfaction, emotional factors, adversarial relationships, and other potential problems. At any rate, assurance of patients' rights is an important element of psychosocial aspects of rehabilitation, but the issue is by no means uncomplicated, as depicted very well by Lipsitt.[98] Nonetheless, advocacy movements have indicated, with little equivocation, that

. . . (3) the patient has the right to obtain from his physician complete current information concerning his diagnosis, treatment, and prognosis in terms the patient can be reasonably expected to understand. When it is not advisable to give such information to the patient, the information shall be made available to an appropriate person in his behalf. He has the right to know by name the physician responsible for coordinating his care. (4) The patient has the right to receive from his physician the information necessary to give informed consent prior to the initiation of any procedure or treatment. Except in emergencies, such information necessary for informed consent shall include but not necessarily be limited to specific procedure or treatment, the significant risks involved, and the probable duration of incapacitation. Where significant alternatives for rehabilitation exist, the patient has the right to such information. The patient also has the right to know the name of the person responsible for performing the particular procedure or treatment . . .*

These statements make clear, of course, that patients have a right to know about their condition where therapeutic risk or death is a likely outcome. A major focus of the issue of the patient's right to die or live is upon *who* should participate in making the decision that a patient, in effect, be allowed to exercise this right to die; *why* such a decision should be made; and *how* such a process should be carried out. "Heroic measures" and "extraordinary means" of prolonging life have been a frequent part of the dialogue concerning this topic, although they have often been ill-defined. The so-called "living will," pioneered by California's Natural Death Act of 1976 and legalized in at least a dozen other states, mandates decisions involving the patient, family, physician, lawyer, and clergyman. More recently, the congressionally established President's Commission for the Study of Ethical Problems in Medicine and Biomedical and Behavior Research recommended that decisions to begin or end life-sustaining therapy ultimately lie with patients or their official representatives. The highly complex legal problems of living wills have been addressed by Raber.[99]

A related consideration is the medical-legal-ethical definition of death, be it "respiratory death" (the patient has stopped breathing), "cardiac death" (a patient's heart has stopped), or "brain death" (as indicated by flat brain waves). Many times, acute situations are encountered in which little time is left to involve anyone else in the decision to extend the person's life or not; likewise, the patient's emotional state at the time may be transitional, and, given a return of the ability to participate rationally in a decision, the patient might well take a position diametrically opposed to one he or she might assume under stress or in a state of temporary "incompe-

*Reprinted from Policy Concerning Patients' Rights and Responsibilities, Gaylord Hospital, Wallingford, Conn., 1982. Used by permission.

tence." Consequently, the potential "lifesaver" on the acute situation scene, often a nurse or doctor in a hospital, makes the decision alone.

Perhaps a more important aspect of this issue to consider is whether life should be supported when it appears to lack "meaningfulness" for the patient and the family. The *quality of life* is a crucial variable in deciding whether life should be extended in the relatively near future. Whether a patient should receive a tracheostomy is, of course, a crucial consideration in this regard, again one that necessarily involves a variety of significant others in contact with the patient. If a tracheostomy preserves the patient's life, but increases his or her suffering and has no prospect of facilitating a meaningful existence, then perhaps medical procedures supporting life should not be applied in the first place. To quote from Brauer,[100] a physician,

Scientific progress has made it possible to delay the outcome of much terminal illness and to alleviate many of the accompanying physical discomforts, yet, paradoxically, because of this very scientific advance, man rarely dies with dignity, in the comfort of his own home, surrounded by his family and friends gathered to pay their last respects. Rather, he is "comforted" by oxygen tanks, tubes in every natural and surgically-made orifice, and busy hospital personnel intent on carrying out the physician's orders. Gone, too, is the comforting archaic custom of being accompanied to the sepulcher by all his prized possessions including, in some cultures, his wife. . . . In our present culture, we need to focus our efforts on achieving psychological support for the patient with a diagnosis of a terminal illness. To do this requires considerable depth and understanding of what the patient is experiencing.[100]

In summary, then, the issue of the patient's right to die is a complex one, and one that is dealt with most effectively in advance and continuously by those staff directly concerned with treatment of the particular patient. Full participation of the patient and that of the family when possible is a crucial facet of this mutual contract. As with any other "helping" process, it is important for all of us to work with patients and families in this area. To ignore the issue because it is considered too complex, because our own anxieties about death and dying interfere, or because helping to make such decisions smacks of "playing God" is to create a major disservice to patients and families. The guidelines are there for us to reckon with, and it is up to us to put them into practice.

Treatment of the Whole Person

In these and other issues, a psychosocial orientation can play an important role. Through the course of many interviews with patients, the question often arises as to whether the patient has ever considered the possibility that psychosocial factors play an important role in his or her disability. Surprisingly, and sometimes even after 10 or 15 years of medical treatment, it is often found that no professional had previously queried this possibility with many patients. This therapeutic approach depicts a rather narrow preoccupation with only the pulmonary system and its malfunctioning. In this situation, one becomes rather quickly convinced that anxiety may be as significant a factor in the patient's disability as the actual disease itself. For example, laboratory physiologic studies might reveal that a particular patient should be able to function at a reasonably higher level. However, in actuality, this patient may be severely disabled as a result of his or her anxiety and inability to cope with illness. Thus, failure to take into account the nonmedical areas of a person's being gives lip service to the concept of the "whole person," to which all of us have been more than casually exposed in our training. A person is therefore treated as a "pair of lungs" without regard to the other important areas in life. Regrettably, allegiance to the traditional medical model may continue even when the predominant problems for the patient and family are emotional, intellectual, interpersonal, social, occupational, and sexual—in short, psychosocial.

Behavioral Techniques

Within an alternative rehabilitation model, preventive and therapeutic interventions, particularly self-regulatory procedures, are based on learning principles. Behavior modification techniques may be used, notably progressive relaxation, in an effort to reduce anxiety, a learned response. More recently, biofeedback (Chapter 7) has been used either independently or in combination with relaxation training with excellent results, thus interrupting the vicious cycle of anxiety followed by dyspnea/followed by anxiety/followed by increase in dyspnea and so on. In addition, yoga, movement therapy, physical therapy, meditation, hypnosis, autogenic training, and guided imagery are helpful in reducing the debilitating effect of pulmonary disease. Of course, individual, group, couple, and family psychotherapy have been on the scene for some time representing effective psychological interventions.

An example of the successful application of psychological techniques in pulmonary rehabilitation is the case of a woman, now 71, who has had a diagnosis of COLD for 20 years. At present she also has the usual associated ailments such as cor pulmonale, arteriosclerotic heart disease, and osteoporotic spinal degeneration as a result of many years of corticosteroid use. Ten years ago, she entered into a training program primarily involving progressive relaxation. Subsequently, her program included guided imagery, specifically to control angina. The description of the pain she experienced and the application of behavioral strategies is depicted in Figure 10–2.

The Pain

Pressure begins in the area under the breastbone corresponding to the heart, an "attack" that cannot be brushed off, because it takes over immediately. This is nearly always followed by severe pain that builds in intensity and spreads outward to the shoulder and left arm and upward to the throat, jaw, and base of the tongue. Initially, there is a pronounced tingling of the fingers of the left hand followed by a continuation of the arm pain as though it were running along a wire to the fingers. The hand is clenched, making it numb, and it is difficult to open a small pill bottle without dropping it.

Initiation of Self-Treatment

The person ingests one nitroglycerin tablet (1/150th mg), which requires 1 to 3 minutes to produce a noticeable reduction in the pain. As soon as possible, instant relaxation is applied throughout the body ("go loose everywhere"), with particular concentration in the specific areas of pain/pressure. Breathing is carefully monitored in conjunction with relaxation, with exhalations twice as long in duration as inhalations. ("Get the old air OUT—the fresh air will rush without effort into the vacuum thus created.")

Visual Imagery

A large metal spike is visualized pressing on the chest region (see illustration below). For varying intervals, 10 seconds to perhaps 30 seconds to 1 minute, only pressure is felt. The pain starts at the point of the spike, rapidly expanding and tearing surrounding tissue. The pain intensifies as the spike gorws hotter and redder. As the pain begins to radiate, this "ramrod" acquires a flaming aura with red-blue-green-violet colors. This spike is supported by all the muscles and tendons through which it has driven. To disarm the spike, cool air is "blown" at it through inhalation. Regular, deep, rhythmic breathing is established, and the scorched muscles grow limp and loose and are thus unable to support the heavy spike. It loses its red-hot color and gradually shrinks, turns dark gray, and ceases to drive inward. In other words, there is a "letting go," and the rod becomes harmless and retires in defeat.

Fig 10–2.—Relaxation and visualization to inhibit angina pain: imagery of spike piercing skin.

Many similar examples could be cited in which progressive relaxation (sometimes provided through group training) provides a foundation for more sophisticated techniques involving imagery, thought-blocking, and covert methods such as sensitization, desensitization, and reinforcement. These are individualized, often adjunctive to psychotherapy, and are designed to provide the patient (and family in many instances) with more effective coping mechanisms within a stress management system.

Sexuality and Disability

Any effective discussion of sexuality and disability, including that pertaining to chronic respiratory insufficiency, must begin with a description of sexuality. Sexuality refers to a deep and pervasive aspect of a person's existence. It is the way we think and feel about ourselves and the way we relate to others—men and women, adults, and children. In a philosophic statement, the Long Range Planning Committee of the American Association of Sex Educators, Counselors and Therapists has stated, "Sex is a natural function, a significant part, but not all, of sexuality. Sexuality includes somatic, emotional, intellectual, social and ethical dimensions of life and constitutes a significant portion of every individual's personality."[101] Sex and sexual functioning are thus an important part of life, an activity of daily living if you will, for most people, and various impairments may create some difficulties in this area. Dyspnea, bronchospasm, altered physical condition, fatigability, and attendant affective states such as anxiety and depression may be factors in this regard. The effects of the impairment are determined by the nature and extent of the disease process. There are also varying individual reactions that must be taken into account in assessing a person's ability to function sexually.

Assuming that sexual function has been altered and that the affected person and his/her partner intend to engage in sexual activities, communication between them is extremely important, even more so than when a disability is not a factor. An understanding of some anatomy and physiology is helpful, as is knowledge of the individualized effects of medication on sexual functioning. Indeed, although it may be overstating a point, even aspirin might be suspect regarding the individualized, sometimes paradoxic, effects upon a person's functioning, including the sexual aspect. Openness to trying new techniques may also be involved in the goal of bringing about pleasure and mutual satisfaction. Learning about the particular disability as it relates to sexual function may be facilitated through reading, viewing audiovisual materials, discussions with other disabled people, and counseling with a professional trained in this area.

Pulmonary disability does not render a man or a woman or child sexless, regardless of age or sexual preference. Understanding one's sexuality is one key to the process of facilitating readaptation within the home and community. In other words, there is more to sexuality than sex.

Although significant strides have been taken in advancing the subject of human sexuality in both public and scientific/professional arenas, mid-Victorian thought still very often prevails. Unfortunately, in our society, it is widely assumed that in order to be "naturally" interested in and capable of enjoying sexual experiences, one must be young, attractive, able-bodied, and heterosexual. It follows, then, that when one has a disability, especially a visible one, and particularly when one is a member of the older segment of the population, others believe that the realm of sexual matters is beyond his or her interest and/or capability. Such a belief is based on several of the following myths, derived from a variety of sources, the exact origin(s) of which are unknown. These myths must be dispelled at nearly every turn when working with persons with disabilities.

The first of these myths is that disabled persons are asexual; that is, that because of actual physical impairments and the tremendous energy invested in adapting, the person is not only unable to participate in meaningful sexual activity, but also is simply not interested. In other words, the major interest in such a person's life is to adapt to the disability. While it is certainly true that issues of life and death and regaining some semblance of health may prevail over and supersede sex for a time, thoughts and feelings about sex do not vanish even when not dealt with directly by the professional.

Other common myths are that the person with a disability is oversexed and has uncontrollable urges or that he or she is dependent and child-like and thus needs to be protected. These myths are primarily fostered by professionals who adopt a condescending manner with patients, as though they have a magical view of what is really happening in the patient's life. Another myth worthy of dispelling is that an erection is necessary for sexual satisfaction. This is an area where culture has placed a tremendous burden on the male. In order to satisfy a partner, an erection is presumably a necessary part of the sexual apparatus. The spinal cord injury literature and clinical experience particularly indicate that this is simply not so.

In the same vein, females have had an increasing burden placed upon them over the past several years, resting on the notion that orgasms are necessary for sexual satisfaction. Indeed, no recent topic in human sexuality has been so heavily researched and discussed as this one, to the extent that a woman who achieves only one orgasm during sex is somehow considered deficient or lacking. Like other myths, this is sheer nonsense. Moreover, even genital intercourse is not necessary for sexual satisfaction.

Finally, other myths that prevail in the mind of not only the public, but, unfortunately, in professionals as well are that disabled persons almost always have sexual problems, that sexual problems are almost always due to the disability, and that sexual problems go away of their own accord. Although pulmonary disability, for example, can create problems in the sexual area, there is no evidence to indicate that patients with chronic respiratory insufficiency experience any more or less problems than the general public. However, if sexual problems prevailed before the onset of the disability, it is quite likely that these problems will be exacerbated afterwards and, without some type of effective professional intervention, will not simply vanish.

Thus, it is important to stress the following general notions:

1. Sexuality cannot be taken away. It is a basic human characteristic that is not earned through work or lost by accident, injury, or illness.

2. Ignorance, as opposed to knowledge and information, is a major deterrent to adaptation to a pulmonary disability.

3. It is important for us as professionals to help clients assume responsibility for their own lives, including the sexual aspect.

4. We can do this by developing *askable* staff in our health care systems who are knowledgeable about sexuality and disability and who are available to discuss sexual matters with their clients.

Viewing sexuality, then, as an activity of daily living, our clients have the right to (1) sexual expression, (2) privacy, (3) be informed, (4) have access to needed services, (5) use avenues of personal decision making, and (6) the development of one's fullest potential.

The writings of Kravetz[102, 103] represent a significant departure from the norm of silence in the area of sex and COLD. He describes the reluctance on the part of both the physician (which can be expanded to include all health professionals) and the patient to discuss the subject because of training deficiencies and taboos. The same lack of attention is shown in the literature, with only a dozen or so articles in existence pertaining to the topic.

Kravetz[103] describes the "emasculation" and loss of virility that occurs in males and a felt decline in female sexual attractiveness associated with lung disease. More importantly, he focuses on the compromise in intimacy as a result. "When the intimacy in a loving relationship is plundered by COLD, the partnership dissolves and becomes a simple association—two people occupying the same space and coping less and less effectively with the unrelenting tensions of chronic disease."[103] This further reinforces the social isolation of the patient with COLD by creating a painful distance between partners, often within the home itself. Kravetz adds: "In a disease marked by isolation and depression, moments of physical, spiritual and emotional closeness with another can outweigh hours of solitary reflection on disability."[102]

Kravetz[102, 103] recommends and this author supports the adoption of Annon's[104–106] PLISSIT Model (an acronym for "permission giving, limited information, specific suggestions, and intensive therapy," useful in office practice). However, this model has potentially effective application within most settings, including institutional ones. Another useful tool recommended is a three-part audiotape/slide presentation that depicts office counseling with male and female patients. This package, produced by Kravetz,[103] is also helpful in professional education.

In addition to the dearth of articles, neglect of the topic of sexuality and pulmonary disease is illustrated by an article published barely 11 years ago.[108] Though important, this publication hardly generated a raft of publications in the field. Sexuality and disability as a field has grown considerably during this period of time, but the application to pulmonary disability has been lacking.

Later articles have been written that have helped raise the consciousness of physicians dealing with pulmonary patients, but have often focused almost exclusively on the male.[108-111] Others, much to their credit, have dealt with the implications of chronic respiratory disease for psychosexual and psychosocial development in children and youth,[112, 113] an area which is even more underrepresented in the literature on sexuality and disability. Evans and Conine[113] urge respiratory therapists to play an active role in promoting sexual health with parents and their children who have COLD, bronchial asthma, or cystic fibrosis. Being informed, providing education and appropriate modeling, and maintaining a positive attitude are features involved in helping families deal with respiratory problems throughout the developmental life span.[113, 114]

In a distinguished article based on a presentation at the 38th annual meeting of the American Geriatrics Society, Masters and Johnson[115] point out that *ageism* in our society tends to suppress appropriate sexual expression and continued effective sexual adjustment among the elderly. They caution that myths and misconceptions cause withdrawal and isolation from intimacy instead of fostering attitudes that continue to give full value to a natural physiologic process. Without alluding specifically to the possible interfering effects of a pulmonary disability, Masters and Johnson discuss two clinical syndromes associated with the aging process, the "Widow's and Widower's Syndromes." These maladies develop following extended periods of no sexual interaction. Mentioning the popular doggerel of "use it or lose it," Masters and Johnson state that ". . . neither aging men nor women can afford long continued periods of coital continence if they are to continue as physically effective sexual partners." This statement needs to be underscored, because a significant portion of COLD patients are elderly and thus are unnecessarily at risk for sexual dysfunction.

Summary

Understanding the impact of a pulmonary disability on the patient and family is a complex but essential process. The patient/family personality affects the response to treatment in any facility as well as on an outpatient basis. Short- and long-term life goals of the patient may be seriously altered regardless of age, sex, education, socioeconomic status, occupation, and marital situation. The psychological experience of hospitalization particularly plays a crucial role in rehabilitation. The patient's perception of the disability may be discrepant with that of the family and/or the staff who work with him or her. Such discrepancies need resolution in the interest of patient care. It is extremely important to understand how the system of delivery of services to the patient actually affects him or her. Often, treatment is subject to external influence by the family, friends, consultants, and/or hospital administration. Interpersonal relationships such as these play a key role in the adjustment the patient makes within a program. The patient, family, staff, and administration must coordinate their efforts in mutual decision making and implementation based on the *needs* of the patient.

As an example of health professionals delivering comprehensive care, respiratory therapists can play a crucial role in the facilitation of rehabilitation by avoiding the role of functioning as a technician only. Unfortunately, an inordinate amount of time in training and education in this field is spent on anatomy and physiology, chemistry, physics, pharmacology, pathology (disease states), emergency/acute care, infection control, pulmonary function testing, continued ventilatory support, gas therapy, and other important *technical* aspects. However, recognizing the importance of the respiratory therapist in the patient's overall perception of his/her treatment, the amount of time therapists spend with the patient, and the potential healing power within the person himself, the therapist can make an even more valuable contribution to patient care. This is often a professional role for which they have not been trained and one that is not particularly easy to carry out, but it nonetheless represents a major step forward for both pulmonary rehabilitation and the profession of respiratory therapy itself, as well as the professions of nursing and occupational and physical therapy.

The antecedents of pulmonary disability may be based either on reversible or reactive changes in the pulmonary system or on nonreversible, anatomic, structural changes. The consequences of these alterations are then dependent on three basic systems:

1. The interaction of the patient with his or her physical environment.

2. Social interaction with those significant others and treating personnel in contact with the patient.

3. The transactional result of all the varied interactions involved in the

disability and the therapeutic intervention(s) developed to help the patient/family cope.

The respiratory therapist and other allied health professionals are thus in a position to make a significant impact on the psychosocial aspects of pulmonary rehabilitation.

In conclusion, when a person has emphysema, bronchitis, asthma, or lung cancer, the resultant medical problems can seriously disrupt his or her life and the lives of the people nearby. Many of the predominant problems the patient and family face are not of a strictly medical nature, but rather are emotional, intellectual, interpersonal, social, occupational, and sexual—in short, psychosocial. The person may be overwhelmed by anxiety due to the uncertainty of the future, angry at the "injustice" of what is occurring, or depressed at the prospect of changing one's life. Such feelings can interfere greatly with the relationships one has with family and friends, to the extent that isolation and withdrawal may develop. Being less active, learning to pace oneself, and no longer working all create sources of stress for the individual and family.

The process of adaptation includes survival from acute exacerbations, regaining some semblance of health, and then rehabilitation. This process emphasizes learning and aims toward a minimum reduction of autonomy, an increased effectiveness of communication, and an active participation by the patient and family in the process, especially with respect to decision making. Adaptation involves coping and mastery and understanding not what functions are lost, but rather what are left, and not what the patient cannot do, but rather how the patient can do what he or she did previously, albeit perhaps differently. Often people faced with drastically altered living circumstances find it helpful to talk with professionals and peers about the areas that concern them. This may involve individual sessions with the patient or couple therapy with the patient and partner, or the entire family may be included if this is the most helpful modality. Individual sessions with any of the family members may also be in order. Group therapy and self-help support groups can also be useful. Facilitation of the rehabilitation process is thus based upon a philosophy of the "whole person," not just a "pair of lungs." These interventions are all designed to assist the patient in reformulating his or her self-concept based on worth rather than on being a defective or deficient person.

References

1. Leigh D.: Some psychiatric aspects of asthma. *Practitioner* 170:381–402, 1953.
2. Dunbar F.: *Emotions and Bodily Changes: A Survey of Literature on Psychosomatic Interrelationships, 1910-1953*, ed. 4. New York, Columbia University Press, 1954.

3. Freeman E.H., Feingold B.F., Schlesinger K., Gorman F.J.: et al.: Psychological variables in allergic disorders: A review. *Psychosom. Med.* 26:543–575, 1964.
4. Turnbull J.W.: Asthma conceived as a learned response. *J. Psychosom. Res.* 6:59–68, 1962.
5. Graham D.T., Lundy R.M., Benjamin L.S., et al.: Specific attitudes in initial interview with patients having different "psychosomatic" diseases. *Psychosom. Med.* 24:257–262, 1962.
6. Ring F.O.: Testing the validity of personality profiles in psychosomatic illnesses. *Am. J. Psychiatry* 113:1075–1084, 1957.
7. Dirks J.F., Fross K.H., Evans N.W.: Panic-fear in asthma: Generalized personality trait vs. specific situational state. *J. Asthma Res.* 14:161–167, 1977.
8. Dahlem N.W., Kinsman R.A., Horton D.J.: Panic-fear in asthma: Requests for as-needed medications in relation to pulmonary function measurements. *J. Allergy Clin. Immunol.* 60:295–300, 1977.
9. Dirks J.F., Kinsman R.A., Horton D.J., et al.: Panic-fear in asthma: Rehospitalization following intensive long-term treatment. *Psychosom. Med.* 40:5–13, 1978.
10. Dirks J.F., Kinsman R.A., Jones N.F., Fross K.H.: New development in panic-fear research in asthma: Validity and stability of the MMPI panic-fear scale. *Br. J. Med. Psychol.* 51:119–126, 1978.
11. Dirks J.F., Kleiger J.H., Evans N.W.: ASC panic-fear and length of hospitalization in asthma. *J. Asthma Res.* 15:95–97, 1978.
12. Dirks J.F., Fross K.H., Paley A.: Panic-fear in asthma—state-trait relationship and rehospitalization. *J.Chronic. Dis.* 31:605–609, 1978.
13. Heller A.S., Dirks J.F.: The effects of patient personality on chronic obstructive pulmonary disease. *J. Am. Soc. Psychosom. Dent. Med.* 25:144–149, 1978.
14. Dirks J.F., Paley A., Fross K.H.: Panic-fear research in asthma and the nuclear conflict theory of asthma: Similarities, differences and clinical implications. *Br. J. Med. Psychol.* 52:71–76, 1979.
15. Dirks J.F., Kinsman R.A., Staudenmayer H., Kleiger J.H.: Panic-fear in asthma: Symptomatology as an index of signal anxiety and personality as an index of ego resources. *J. Nerv. Ment. Dis.* 167:615–619, 1979.
16. Jones N.F., Kinsman R.A., Dirks J.F., Dahlem N.W.: Psychological contributions to chronicity in asthma: Patient response styles influencing medical treatment and its outcome. *Med. Care.* 17:1103–1118, 1979.
17. Dirks J.F., Jones N.F., Fross K.H.: Psychosexual aspects of the panic-fear personality types in asthma. *Can. J. Psychiatry* 24:731–739, 1979.
18. Kinsman R.A., Dirks J.F., Dahlem N.W., Heller A.S.: Anxiety in asthma: Panic-fear symptomatology and personality in relation to manifest anxiety. *Psychol. Rep.* 46:196–198, 1980.
19. Kinsman R.A., Dirks J.F., Jones N.F.: Levels of psychological experience in asthma: General and illness-specific concomitants of panic-fear personality. *J. Clin. Psychol.* 36:552–561, 1980.
20. Fross K.H., Dirks J.F., Kinsman R.A., Jones N.F.: Functionally determined invalidism in chronic asthma. *J. Chronic Dis.* 33:485–490, 1980.
21. Dirks J.F., Schraa J.C., Brown E.L., Kinsman R.A.: Psychomaintenance in asthma: Hospitalization rates and financial impact. *Br. J. Med. Psychol.* 53:349–354, 1980.

22. Dirks J.F., Kinsman R.A.; Clinical prediction of medical hospitalization: Psychological assessment with the battery of asthma illness behavior. *J. Pers. Assess.* 45:608–613, 1981.

23. Dirks J.F., Robinson S.K., Dirks D.L.: Alexithymia and the psychomaintenance of bronchial asthma. *Psychother. Psychosom.* 36:63–71, 1981.

24. Dirks J.F., Kinsman R.A.: Bayesian prediction of noncompliance: As-needed (PRN) medication usage patterns and the battery of asthma illness behavior. *J. Asthma Res.* 19:25–31, 1982.

25. Dirks J.F.: Bayesian prediction of psychomaintenance related to rehospitalizations in asthma. *J. Pers. Assess.* 46:159–163, 1982.

26. Hudgel D.W., Cooperson D.M., Kinsman R.A.: Recognition of added loads in asthma: The importance of behavioral styles. *Am. Rev. Respir. Dis.* 126:121–125, 1982.

27. Kaptein A.A.: Psychological correlates of length of hospitalization and rehospitalization in patients with acute, severe asthma. *Soc. Sci. Med.* 16:725–729, 1982.

28. Lebowitz M.D., Thompson H.C., Strunk R.C.: Subjective psychological symptoms in outpatient asthmatic adolescents. *J. Behav. Med.* 4:439–449, 1981.

29. Matus I.: Assessing the nature and clinical significance of psychological contribution to childhood asthma. *Am. J. Orthopsychiatry* 51:327–341, 1981.

30. Staudenmayer H.: Medical manageability and psychosocial factors in childhood asthma. *J. Chronic Dis.* 35:183–198, 1982.

31. Abramson H.A., Peshkin M.M.: Psychosomatic group therapy with parents of children with intractable asthma: XI. The Goldey family, part I. *J. Asthma Res.* 17:31–47, 1979.

32. _____: XII. _____, part 2. *J. Asthma Res.* 17:81–99, 180.

33. _____: XIII. _____, part 3. *J. Asthma Res.* 17:123–147, 1980.

34. Wilson C.P.: Parental overstimulation in asthma. *Int. J. Psychoanal. Psychother.* 8:601–621, 1980-81.

35. Groen J.J.: The psychosomatic theory of bronchial asthma. *Psychother. Psychosom.* 31:38–48, 1979.

36. Rutter B.M.: Measurement of psychological factors in chronic illness. *Rheumatol. Rehabil.* 15:174–178, 1976.

37. Rutter B.M.: Some psychological concomitants of chronic bronchitis. *Psychol. Med.* 7:459–464, 1977.

38. Rutter B.M.: The prognostic significance of psychological factors in the management of chronic bronchitis. *Psychol. Med.* 9:63–70, 1979.

39. *Cancer Facts and Figures.* New York, American Cancer Society, 1983.

40. *Make Cancer Control Your Business.* New York, American Cancer Society, 1981.

41. Gordon W.A., Freidenbergs I., Diller L., et al.: Efficacy of psychosocial intervention with cancer patients. *J. Consult. Clin. Psychol.* 48:743–759, 1980.

42. Achterberg J., Lawlis G.F., Simonton O.C., Matthews-Simonton S.: Psychological factors and blood chemistries as disease outcome predictors for cancer patients. *Multivariate Exper. Clin. Res.* 3:107–122, 1977.

43. Winder A.E.: Family therapy: A necessary part of the cancer patient's care: A multidisciplinary treatment concept. *Family Ther.* 5:151–161.

44. Wortman C.B., Dunkel-Schetter C.: Interpersonal relationships and cancer: A theoretical analysis. *J. Soc. Issues* 5:120–154, 1979.

45. Shanfield S.B.: On surviving cancer: Psychological considerations. *Compr. Psychiatry* 21:128–134, 1980.
46. Giaquinta B.: Helping families face the crisis of cancer. *Am. J. Nurs.* 77:1585–1588, 1977.
47. Kimbel P., Kaplan A.S., Alkalax I., Lester D.: An inhospital program for rehabilitation of patients with chronic obstructive pulmonary disease. *Chest* 60(suppl.):65–105, 1971.
48. Neff T.A., Petty T.L.: Outpatient care for patients with chronic airway obstruction, emphysema and bronchitis. *Chest* 60(suppl.):115S–175S, 1971.
49. Farrington J.F.: Rehabilitation of pulmonary cripple in private practice. *Chest* 60(suppl.):185S–205S, 1971.
50. Matzen R.N.: Vocational rehabilitation—the culmination of physical reconditioning. *Chest* 60(suppl.):215S–245S, 1971.
51. Care in respiratory disease, in *Nursing Clinics of North America*, vol. 9. Philadelphia, W.B. Saunders Co., 1974.
52. Kimbel P.: Physical therapy for COPD patients. *Clin. Notes Respir. Dis.*, vol. 8, 1970.
53. Proceedings of the Conference on the Scientific Basis of In-Hospital Respiratory Therapy. *Am. Rev. Respir. Dis.*, vol. 5, 1980.
54. Berzins G.F.: An occupational therapy program for the chronic obstructive pulmonary disease patient. *Am. J. Occup. Ther.* 24:181–186, 1970.
55. Pomerantz P., Flannery E.L., Findling P.K.: Occupational therapy for chronic obstructive lung disease. *Am. J. Occup. Ther.* 29:181–186, 1970.
56. Pierce J.A.: Office management of chronic obstructive pulmonary disease. *Clin. Notes Respir. Dis.*, vol. 7, 1968.
57. Fishman D.B., Petty T.L.: Physical, symptomatic and psychological improvement in patients receiving comprehensive care for chronic airway obstruction. *J. Chronic Dis.* 24:775–785, 1971.
58. Dudley D.L., Wermuth C., Hague W.: Psychosocial aspects of care in the chronic obstructive pulmonary disease patient. *Heart Lung* 2:349–393, 1973.
59. Backus F.I., Dudley D.L.: Observations of psychosocial factors and their relationship to organic disease. *Int. J. Psychiatry Med.* 5:449–515, 1974.
60. Dudley D.L.: Coping with chronic COPD: Therapeutic options. *Geriatrics* 36:69–74, 1981.
61. Dudley D.L., Glaser E.M., Jorgenson B.N., Logan D.L.: Psychosocial concomitants to rehabilitation in chronic obstructive pulmonary disease: I. Psychosocial and psychological considerations. *Chest* 77:413–420, 1980.
62. _____: II. Psychosocial treatment. *Chest* 77:544–551, 1980.
63. _____: III. Dealing with psychiatric disease (as distinguished from psychosocial or psychophysiological problems). *Chest* 77:677–684, 1980.
64. Dudley D.L., Pitts-Poarch A.R.: Psychophysiological aspects of respiratory control. *Clin. Chest Med.* 1:131–143, 1980.
65. Dudley D.L., Sitzman J.: Psychosocial and psychophysiologic approach to the patient. *Semin. Respir. Med.* 1:59–83, 1979.
66. Krop H.D., Block A.J., Cohen E.: Neuropsychologic effects of continuous oxygen therapy in chronic obstructive pulmonary disease. *Chest* 64:317–322, 1973.
67. Krop H.D., Block A.J., Cohen E., et al.: Neuropsychologic effects of continuous oxygen therapy in the aged. *Chest* 72:737–743, 1977.
68. Grant I., Heaton R.K., McSweeny A.J., et al.: Brain dysfunction in COPD. *Chest* 77(suppl.):308–309, 1980.
69. Woolcock A.J.: Conference summary. *Chest* 77(suppl.):326–330, 1980.

70. Vanderpool H.Y.: Health care for the whole person. Paper presented at the American Association for Respiratory Therapy Annual Convention, Oct. 31, 1982.
71. Scoggins W., Simpson K.: Pulmonary rehabilitation. Paper presented at the American Association for Respiratory Therapy Annual Convention, Nov. 2, 1982.
72. Hodgkin J.E. (ed.): *Chronic Obstructive Pulmonary Disease: Current Concepts in Diagnosis and Comprehensive Care.* (Park Ridge, Ill., American College of Chest Physicians, 1979.
73. Haas A., Pineda H., Haas F., Axen K.: *Pulmonary Therapy and Rehabilitation Principles and Practice.* Baltimore, Williams & Wilkins Co., 1979.
74. Strauss A.: *Chronic Disease and the Quality of Life.* St. Louis, C.V. Mosby Co., 1975, pp. 77–79.
75. Agle D.P., Baum G.L.: Psychological aspects of chronic obstructive pulmonary disease. *Med. Clin. North Am.* 61:749–768, 1977.
76. Flanagan J.C.: Measurement of quality of life: Current state of the art. *Arch. Phys. Med. Rehabil.* 63:56–59, 1982.
77. Kottke F.: Philosophic considerations of quality of life for the disabled. *Arch. Phys. Med. Rehabil.* 63:60–62, 1982.
78. Caputi M.: A "quality of life" model for social work practice in health care. *Health Soc. Work* 7:103–110, 1982.
79. McSweeny A.J., Grant I., Heaton R.K., et al.: Life quality of patients with chronic obstructive pulmonary disease. *Arch. Intern. Med.* 142:473–478, 1982.
80. McSweeny A.J., Heaton R.K., Grant I., et al.: Chronic obstructive pulmonary disease: Socioemotional adjustment and life quality. *Chest* 77(suppl.):309–311, 1980.
81. Seiler L.H.: Final Report: The Fifteen-Month Patient Education Study. New York, American Lung Association, 1979.
82. Post L., Collins C.: The poorly coping COPD patient: A psychotherapeutic perspective. *Int. J. Psychiatry Med.* 11:173–182, 1981–82.
83. Bowen W.T., Marler D.C., Androes L.: The psychiatric team: Myth and mystique. *Am. J. Psychiatry* 122:687–690, 1965.
84. Katz A., Bender E. (eds.): *The Strength in Us: Self-Help Groups in the Modern World.* New York, Franklin Watts, 1976.
85. Evans G.: *The Family Circle Guide to Self-Help.* New York, Ballantine Books, 1979.
86. *Hospital Involvement with Self-Help/Support Groups.* Chicago, American Hospital Association, Center for Health Promotion, 1981.
87. *Plain Talk About Mutual Help Groups.* Washington, D.C., National Institute of Mental Health, Division of Scientific and Public Information, 1981.
88. Gartner A., Riessman F.: *Help: A Working Guide to Self-Help Groups.* New York, New Viewpoints-Vision Books, 1980.
89. Gussow A., Tracy G.: Role of self-help clubs in adaptation to chronic illness and disability. *Soc. Sci. Med.* 10:407–414, 1976.
90. Lieberman M., Borman L. (eds.): *Self-Help Groups for Coping With Crisis.* San Francisco, Jossey-Bass, Inc., 1979.
91. Gartner A.J., Riessman F.: Self-help and mental health. *Hosp. Community Psychiatry* 33:631–635, 1982.
92. Durman E.C.: The role of self-help in service provision. *J. Appl. Behav. Sci.* 12:433–443, 1976.
93. DeMocker J.D., Zimpfer D.G.: Group approaches to psychosocial interven-

tion in medical care: A synthesis. *Int. J. Group Psychother.* 31:247–260, 1981.
94. Romanik K. (ed.): *Around the Clock with COPD.* Wallingford, Conn., Gaylord Respiratory Club, 1982.
95. Golodetz A., Ruess J., Milhous R.L.: The right to know: Giving the patient his medical record. *Arch. Phys. Med. Rehabil.* 57:78–81, 1976.
96. Stevens D.P., Stagg R., MacKay I.: What happens when hospitalized patients see their own records. *Ann. Intern. Med.* 86:474–477, 1977.
97. Altman J.H., Reich P., Kelly M.J., Rogers M.P.: Patients who read their medical charts. *N. Engl. J. Med.* 302:169–171, 1980.
98. Lipsitt D.R.: The patient and the record. *New Engl. J. Med.* 302:167–168, 1980.
99. Raber P.E.: Ethical and legal problems of living wills. *Geriatrics* 35:27–30, 1980.
100. Brauer P.H.: Should the patient be told the truth? *Nurs. Outlook,* vol. 8, 1960.
101. Long Range Planning Committee, American Association of Sex Educators, Counselors and Therapists: *AASECT Newsletter* 13(4), December 1982.
102. Kravetz H.M.: Sexual counseling for the COPD patient. *Clin. Challenge in Cardiopul. Med.* 4(1):1–5, 1982.
103. Kravetz H.M.: Sexual counseling of the COPD patient. *Continuing Education* November 1982, pp. 47–50.
104. Annon J.S.: The PLISSIT model: A proposed conceptual scheme for the behavioral treatment of sexual problems. *J. Sex Educ. Ther.* 2:1–15, 1976.
105. Annon J.S.: *The Behavioral Treatment of Sexual Problems.* Honolulu, Enabling Systems, Inc., 1976.
106. Pion P., Annon J.S.: The office management of sexual problems: Brief therapy approaches. *J. Reprod. Med.* 15:127–144, 1975.
107. Plummer J.K. Developing an institutional program in sexuality and disability: Sociopolitical considerations, programmatic aspects. Paper presented at the Annual Meeting of the American Associaton of Sex Educators, Counselors and Therapists, New York City, 1982; at the Fourth Annual National Symposium on Sexuality and Disability, New York City, 1982; and at the Burke Conference on Sexuality and Disability, White Plains, 1983.
108. Kass I., Updegraff K., Muffly R.B.: Sex in chronic obstructive pulmonary disease. *Med. Aspects Hum. Sexual.* 6:33–42, 1972.
109. Straus S., Dudley D.L.: Sexual activity for asthmatics—a psychiatric perspective. *Med. Aspects Hum. Sexual.* 10:63–64, 1976.
110. Lyons H.A.: Sexual relations for male patients with chronic obstructive lung disease. *Med. Aspects Hum. Sexual.* 11:119–120, 1977.
111. Fletcher E.C., Martin R.J.: Sexual dysfunction and erectile impotence in chronic obstructive pulmonary disease. *Chest* 81:113–121, 1982.
112. Taussig L.M., Cohen M., Sieber O.F.: Psychosexual and psychosocial aspects of cystic fibrosis. *Practitioner* 224:301–303, 1980.
113. Evans J.H., Conine T.A.: Development of sexuality in children with chronic obstructive pulmonary disease. *Respir. Care* 27:687–692, 1982.
114. Conine T.A., Evans J.H.: Sexual adjustment in chronic obstructive pulmonary disease. *Respir. Care* 26:871–874, 1981.
115. Masters W.H., Johnson V.E.: Sex and the aging process. *J. Am. Geriatr. Soc.* 29:385–390, 1981.

11 / Patient Education

TALI A. CONINE, D.H.S., R.P.T.

REHABILITATION REFERS to a process aimed at restoring a person to useful life "through education and therapy."[1] Pulmonary rehabilitation therefore involves care giving and patient education with the objective of promoting independence, physical health, and emotional comfort. The teaching-learning process is central to effective rehabilitation, and teaching skills are prominent in the quality of service provided by therapists, nurses, and other professionals.

Rehabilitation personnel explain many things to patients and attempt to help them develop certain skills and habits. When a patient is "taught," the experienced therapist knows that he cannot necessarily assume that learning has taken place. Several basic questions are implicit in learning:

1. What is expected to be accomplished, or what are the objectives of teaching?

2. Does the patient want to learn?

3. What is the best way to teach?

4. How does the therapist know whether or not the patient has learned? This chapter will focus on the process of patient teaching and learning, and will briefly address each of the above questions.

The Objectives Of Patient Education

The opportunity for teaching in rehabilitation presents itself in a number of ways. A patient or a family member may ask a direct question such as, "Why is the color of my sputum sometimes pink after using the nebulizer?" A physician may refer a patient with a request: "Teach the patient how to use the hand-held nebulizer." The need for teaching may become apparent while observing the patient. For example, in a predischarge teaching situation, the therapist may notice that the capillary tube of the nebulizer is probably clogged, but notes the patient does not make the same observation. Though these and other situations may be frequently repeated in pulmonary rehabilitation, the goals and objectives of teaching must vary with each individual. The reasons for variation are several, including the person's desire or level of motivation to learn, his health beliefs and habits,

173

his educational background and intellectual capabilities, his physical condition, and his environment. Though all of these considerations interrelate, the teaching objectives of a therapist may be categorized into three separate groups or "domains": (1) *affective*, when the purpose is to change patient's attitudes and level of motivation, (2) *cognitive*, when the purpose is to help the patient understand some facts or concepts, and (3) *psychomotor*, when the focus is on teaching manipulative skills and coordinated physical tasks to the patient.

An effective therapist is capable of not only identifying the specific purposes of his teaching (i.e., teaching domains), but he can also communicate them to the patient and other personnel in terms of specific objectives. The example in Table 11–1 illustrates how a therapist may express the manner in which his patient, the learner, is expected to feel (affective domain), think (cognitive domain), and act (psychomotor domain) by the educative process.

Each statement of objective should point out a single patient behavior, in the form of a verb, and a content that would indicate what the patient is to do as a consequence of patient education. It is important that consideration be given to arranging the behaviors to be learned in a sequential manner, from simple to complex, and to the necessary priority for safety and adequate functioning.

Bloom[2] and Krathwohl and associates[3] have defined and listed teaching/learning behaviors in terms of complexity, thereby aiding in communication of purposes regarding teaching and evaluation of learning. To become proficient in stating patient-teaching goals, it is suggested that the therapist read these authors' handbooks and use an excellent self-instructional presentation, *Preparing Instructional Objectives*, by Robert Mager.[4]

In teaching the patient, as in other aspects of professional decision mak-

TABLE 11–1.—EXAMPLE OF PATIENT EDUCATION OBJECTIVES

PURPOSE: TO USE HAND NEBULIZER (SQUEEZE-BULB TYPE)

AFFECTIVE OBJECTIVES	COGNITIVE OBJECTIVES	PSYCHOMOTOR OBJECTIVES
1. To agree that it is desirable.	1. To dilute medicine in 1:3 ratio.	1. To close mouth around mouthpiece.
2. To verbalize willingness to use it.	2. To use 1/2 hr before meals and bedtime.	2. To squeeze the bulb rapidly.
3. To follow instructions and feel satisfaction with results.	3. To recognize causes of mouthpiece malfunction.	3. To inhale slowly and deeply, then hold breath for 2 sec × 4 breaths.
		4. To rinse mouth with water without swallowing.

ing, the therapist continually sets goals even though he may not consciously label them as such. There are three important reasons for formulating and stating the objectives as shown in Table 11–1. The first is to make clear exactly what is to be accomplished. The second is that the statements provide direction and serve as a guide for planning action. The third reason for establishing objectives is that they serve as the key to the evaluation of teaching and learning. These purposes will be discussed in more detail later in this chapter.

Motivation To Learn

Since learning requires that the patient desires to learn, a realistic therapist does not set teaching goals without considering the patient's level of motivation to learn and his willingness to comply with instructions. If a patient shows no interest, a therapist will face a real challenge in discovering the reason for the indifference and in attempting to overcome it. Lack of motivation to learn and failure to adhere to medical regimens are two common sources of treatment failure and concern for professionals. Many of the same persuasive strategies can be effectively used to improve patient motivation to learn as well as his compliance.

Motivation is a drive within an individual that makes him want to do something. It is possible to treat a patient in ways that will encourage him to want to learn. Some motivating principles include the following:

1. The patient's (learner's) motivation is automatically directed toward his most pressing need. A need is a lack of something wanted or deemed desirable by the learner. Maslow has identified physiologic needs as the most basic of all human needs, followed in order of importance by safety, love, esteem, and self-actualization.[5] Lower-level needs must be satisfied before a patient can be concerned with the higher needs. The therapist can help the patient to want to learn by appealing to his desire to get well, to stay well, to be pain-free, to look attractive, to return to work, or whatever is the patient's perceived need and desire. Involving the patient in goal setting serves to identify to the therapist the patient's perception of his needs.

2. Satisfaction and feeling of accomplishment reinforce motivation. The therapist can stimulate learning by first providing easier tasks or situations in which the patient can succeed, making him aware of his achievement (e.g., changes of his physical or physiologic status), giving him encouragement and feedback, and establishing a pleasant environment that is conducive to satisfaction of social-emotional needs.

3. Motivation to learn is enhanced if what is to be learned is clearly understood by the patient. Precise statements of objectives and their communication to the patient are essential to learning. Good organization of

material and equipment, using a variety of learning experiences and audio-visual materials, and relating new tasks to those already known are all techniques that can be used to make information more meaningful and to motivate the patient.

Compliance is the degree to which a patient adheres to a prescribed regimen, such as taking a drug, performing an exercise, keeping appointments, or a combination of these. The noncompliant patient may carry out more or only a part of the prescribed treatment, do more than recommended, or be erratic about the treatment. Patients are more likely to comply if (1) they have a sufficient knowledge of the disease and what is expected of them; (2) they accept their diagnosis and its seriousness; (3) instruction is given to them both verbally and in writing; and (4) they are assigned to specific health professionals (e.g., physician, therapist) at a specific time. Patient education, follow-up letters, telephone calls reminding patients of appointments or instructions, therapists' enthusiasm and rapport with patient and better and faster service are all factors that contribute to patient compliance.[6,7]

No single technique can be consistently successful in dealing with human relations and motivations. The basic ideas and concepts presented here may be selected and applied as most suitable to the needs and the personality of the patient. The underlying principle for getting someone to change certain behaviors, to learn, or to comply is termed *persuasion*. Effective persuasion usually consists of assisting people to see their self-interest. Fear-arousing methods, commonly used by health professionals, do *not* persuade. Fear often generates resentment and grudging compliance that does not last long.

Best Way To Teach

Several time-tested assumptions guide all experienced teachers. The most basic assumption is that no single teaching method or style is suited for all learners. People learn in different ways and speeds as influenced by differences in aptitudes, backgrounds, or motivation levels. The task of the therapist is to accommodate whatever learning assets the patient has by using a variety of instructional strategies, tools, and technologies.

The second assumption is that people learn best by active participation. The disease process and the institutional atmosphere of hospitals tend to place patients in passive roles. Passivity is not conducive to learning. Patients must be *involved* in their own learning by reading, by responding to questions, by manipulating equipment, by keeping charts, by interpreting diagrams, or by whatever means that requires *doing*.

A third assumption is that learning, to be effective, must convey a purpose or target that is "real" for the patient (i.e., relates to his lifestyle). The therapist can achieve his teaching objectives only when he can stand in the patient's shoes, so to speak, and communicate in terms that are understandable, convincing, and consistent with the self-perceived needs, circumstances, and behavior patterns of the patient.

In general, each of the three learning domains responds best to particular methods of teaching. Facts and concepts (cognitive domain) are best taught by the use of written materials, audiovisual aids, explanations of information, feedback on achievement of goals, and discussion. Attitudes (affective domain) can be influenced through providing a role model to imitate and by discussion aimed at gaining the patient's acceptance and insight into his feelings. Group learning can save a therapist a great deal of time for cognitive and affective teaching by creating the opportunity for patients to profit from each other's experiences and to project desirable role models. The group approach, using peer influence, is also a viable method for persuading patients. Motor skills (psychomotor domain) are best learned through demonstration by the health professional, with subsequent practice by the patient until the skills are perfected.

Teaching the Young Learner

Teaching young patients requires special planning and organization. Some basic guidelines include the following:

1. Goals should be geared to a child's level and explained even to 2- to 4-year-olds.

2. Keep messages short, simple, and relayed at eye level. With children below 5 years of age, use fantasy and short stories to give messages.

3. Treat even the young child as a "grown-up," and talk adult-to-adult through both verbal and nonverbal communication.

4. Expect the child to be a responsible and active participant by setting goals, keeping charts or check points, and developing schedules and appointments.

5. Instruction can be followed by a child after the age of 2 years, especially if accompanied by frequent praise, assurance, and realistic feedback.

Evaluation of Patient Education

The crucial question in patient education is, "Has he (the patient) learned what I set out to teach him?" This question emphasizes the essential concept that evaluation is inextricably related to the objectives of teaching, clearly focusing on learning as the end product. Although evaluation is the last step in the process of teaching, it is based on information gathered by various measurement techniques during planning, in actual teaching, and at the conclusion of teaching. During the planning of teaching, evaluation focuses on determining the patient's needs, intellectual ability, and motivation level. This assessment is necessary for formulating sufficiently limited and clearly stated objectives.

Evaluation during teaching serves to reinforce desirable behaviors of the patient and analyze the success or lack of progress made to guide teaching activities. Indications of successful learning may be obtained by the therapist making mental notes of the questions asked by the patient (thus indicating the patient's grasp of the content), the body language of the patient (e.g., a frown or hesitancy), the observation of patient in actual situations performing a demonstrated skill or a desirable attitude, and by asking direct verbal questions or using written quizzes. The evidence gathered during teaching is helpful in assessing whether (1) the objectives are appropriate and possible for the patient to achieve, (2) the principles of learning are consistently being applied, and (3) the communication and level of rapport is effective.

Because learning requires time, practice, and further experiences to be thoroughly assimilated, it is not always possible to determine immediately how well a patient has learned. Allowing for time and practice, final evaluation of cognitive and psychomotor skills is relatively simple through the use of verbal questioning and observation. For example, a patient may be asked why he is preparing equipment in the manner he is. His technique of using the equipment can be simultaneously observed and evaluated. The methods of questioning and observation can be time consuming, but they provide an immediate knowledge of the learner's achievement. In contrast, obtaining a measure of behavior in the affective domain is very difficult and complex. What people say they would do, and what they actually do, may be different. The patient may consciously and subconsciously control the expression of his true feelings. Therefore, the best opportunity for accurate assessment of affective objectives is by observing the patient when he is unaware that he is being observed. Unfortunately, natural behavior is often inaccessible, because it usually occurs in private. The taxonomies of educational objectives[2,3] not only provide a general classification of behaviors, but they may be used also as a guide in considering methods of evaluation of teaching.

Teaching Patients: A Helping Relationship

Teaching is basically a purposeful communication within the context of a helping relationship. The professional is attempting to adapt his scientific knowledge to the needs and backgrounds of the learner. Typically, the individual who suffers from breathing difficulties despairs easily and is anxious about pain, progressive disability, and the threat of death. Fears, helplessness, loneliness, boredom, and dependency may severely interfere with his education and rehabilitation. The competent therapist is acutely aware of the underlying psychological dimensions involved in health care delivery. To facilitate teaching, the therapist uses principles and guidelines from the helping disciplines directly concerned with human interaction, such as counseling, education, psychiatry, and social work. Reaching out to others as a helper depends on one's ability to listen and to respond with the qualities of empathy and warmth. People are not born with these qualities. Skillful interpersonal functioning is learned.[8]

Listening is more than hearing or attending to sounds. Listening is the bridge between hearing and understanding, and is accomplished by grasping the true meaning of not only what is heard, but also what is observed beneath and beyond the surface.[9,10] It requires attending to sound as well as to tone, emphasis, choice of words, silence, gesture, and body language. Observation and listening are inseparable and are imperative to understanding. In a classic book, Bird suggests that the main object of talking to patients should be "to get the patient to talk, to hear from him, to listen."[11] Listening may provide the therapist with an opportunity to learn something new about the patient, to better understand the patient's needs and problems, to establish rapport, and in turn, to encourage the patient to listen more attentively.[9] Table 11–2 provides helpful hints for effective listening in a teaching-helping relationship.

Empathy is the ability to communicate understanding by giving and receiving verbal communication in an atmosphere of warmth and trust. Carkhuff has stated that "without empathy there is no basis for helping."[12] Throughout this chapter and elsewhere in this book, the importance of observation, rapport, communication, feedback, and the ability to look at the world through the patient's eyes have been projected. These qualities are the essential and common ingredients to competent patient care, to a

TABLE 11–2.—THE CHARACTERISTICS OF AN EFFECTIVE LISTENER IN A TEACHING-HELPING RELATIONSHIP

1. Mentally reviews and summarizes what the patient is saying in order to prevent "half-listening."
2. Wonders what the words and phrases mean to the patient, especially if there are differences in their cultural, socioeconomic, ethnic, or educational backgrounds.
3. Looks for nonverbal expressions, such as a grimace or a grasping at the bedclothes.
4. Notes a fall in tone of voice, abrupt silence, shift of topic, contradictions, gaps, repetitions, or unclear meaning and messages.
5. Maintains comforting eye contact (not staring), at similar heights, and close enough to show interest.
6. Reassures the patient of attentiveness by nonverbal cues: leaning forward and toward the patient, appearing at ease, and keeping the arms unfolded.

TABLE 11–3.—The Characteristics of an Empathic Teacher

1. Conveys respect, acceptance, and concern.
2. Focuses on the content *and* feelings being conveyed in message.
3. Interprets for the learner the information that is essential to the treatment or teaching without attempting to impose personal values or beliefs.
4. Identifies options and alternatives.
5. Allows for self-direction and self-choice.
6. Provides encouraging feedback and praise when deserved.
7. Does not threaten, create fear, give advice, or promise greater results than can be reasonably expected.

helping relationship, to a successful exchange of information, and to effective teaching and persuasion. Table 11–3 lists empathic behaviors that would assist the therapist in his teaching role.

Summary

With the establishment of a concept of rehabilitation as a teaching and helping process, the health professional is prepared to develop the skills essential to his care-giving responsibilities. Identifying and stating the teaching objectives, selecting appropriate methods to facilitate learning, assessing patient's needs and progress, and using persuasive strategies are the building blocks in patient education. Fundamental to these tasks is a framework for the provision of service based on a knowledge of human behavior and the principles of effective listening and empathic communication.

References

1. Morris W. (ed.): *The American Heritage Dictionary of the English Language.* Boston, American Heritage Publishing Co., and Houghton Mifflin Co., 1975.
2. Bloom B.S. (ed.): *Taxonomy of Educational Objectives: The Classification of Education Goals.* Handbook 1: *Cognitive Domain.* New York, David McKay Co., 1956.
3. Krathwohl D.R., Bloom B.S., Masian B.B.: *Taxonomy of Educational Objectives: The Classification of Educational Goals.* Handbook II: *Affective Domain.* New York, David McKay Co., 1964.
4. Mager R.F.: *Preparing Instructional Objectives.* Palo Alto, Calif., Fearon Publishers, 1962.
5. Maslow A.H.: A theory of human motivation. *Psychol. Rev.* 50:370–396, 1943.
6. Mayo N.E.: Patient compliance: Practical implications for physical therapists. *Phys. Ther.* 58:1083–1090, 1978.
7. Puckett M.J., Russell M.L.: The role of the allied health professional in improving patient adherence. *J. Allied Health* 7:36–40, 1978.
8. Rubin F.L., Judd M.M., Conine T.A.: Empathy: Can it be learned and retained? *Phys. Ther.* 57:644–647, 1977.

9. Conine T.A.: Listening in the helping relationship. *Phys. Ther.* 56:159–162, 1976.
10. Schulman E.D.: *Intervention in Human Services,* ed. 2. St. Louis, C.V. Mosby Co., 1978, pp. 15–17.
11. Bird B.: *Talking With Patients,* ed. 2. Philadelphia, J.B. Lippincott Co., 1973, p. 10.
12. Carkhuff, R.R.: *Helping and Human Relations,* vol. 2. New York, Holt, Rinehart, & Winston, p. 83.

12 / Starting a Pulmonary Rehabilitation Program

JERRY A. O'RYAN, B.S., R.R.T.

TO DISCUSS THE INITIATION and day-to-day operation of a pulmonary rehabilitation facility is to discuss one of the more pragmatic approaches found in new health care ventures. This simply means that the very newness of the discipline allows a more liberal interpretation of how such an undertaking can be initiated and then operated once it is fully functioning. It is this pioneer spirit that makes the art and science of pulmonary rehabilitation, in both its therapy and medical aspects, rewarding to establish and practice. This chapter should especially be of help to the novice practitioner (physician, respiratory therapist, and those in associated disciplines interested in pulmonary rehabilitation) desiring to initiate a pulmonary rehabilitation program from the ground up or to expand or improve an existing program. This chapter may equally help flourishing programs to assess the qualitative and quantitative values of their present endeavors.

The First Step: Marketing

The first step, and the most important one, is to find out what the physicians referring patients to you perceive pulmonary rehabilitation to be. For example, some physicians may perceive pulmonary rehabilitation as merely a direct extension of the conventional respiratory therapy modalities commonly ordered. They may not be aware of the various and specific components exclusive to this field. Therefore, it is imperative that physicians be made aware of the scope and objectives of pulmonary rehabilitation.

A flow plan is advisable, depicting how patients are entered and how their progress is monitored throughout the entire rehabilitative process. Table 12–1 is one example of a flow plan. Such a chart also helps the physician and others ascertain the general area that the patient is in at any given point in his program.

Table 12–2 is an example of an announcement of the initiation of the program. Marketing of the program at the onset, with regular reminders

182

TABLE 12–1.—SEQUENCE OF PATIENT GOING THROUGH PULMONARY
RECONDITIONING PROGRAM*†

1. Patient is referred by physician's office or via outpatient coordination with Grandview Hospital.
2. First appointment is a pulmonary assessment:
   1. Respiratory history
   2. Pulmonary function
   3. Sputogenesis
   4. Purified protein derivative
   5. Cardiopulmonary stress
   6. X-ray
3. Therapist confers with medical director and referring physician, and final medical advice is obtained.
4. Pulmonary reconditioning program started: basics on diaphragmatic breathing taught, patient given booklet on lung diseases, and range of motion exercises started.
5. Patient learns more of the various range of motion exercises, and walking exercise is started.
6. Treadmill, bicycle, and/or stair climbing exercise is started.
7. Reassessment done at 4 to 6 weeks and pulmonary function repeated; results sent to physician.
8. Based on results of the reassessment, (a) patient continues current regimen of therapy, (b) patient's frequency of visits is decreased, or (c) patient's program is expanded.

*Throughout the patient's reconditioning program, progress reports are sent to the physician. All phases of program are evaluated relative to patient's ability throughout program to obtain maximum reconditioning and increase of pulmonary reserve.
†From Southview Hospital and Family Health Center, Dayton, Ohio.

to the referring physicians, cannot be overstressed. The medical director of the program, usually the physician in charge of respiratory therapy, can greatly assist in diplomatically advertising the program. The cooperation of the support departments need to be fully solicited also, e.g., physical therapy, occupational therapy, dietary, social services, etc.

As time goes by and the program reaches a steady-state point, seminars and more formal written presentations can be developed. Again, a professional marketing approach in all projects is important. Your program will not be given any more serious consideration by those potential users of its service than what your visible marketing attempts appear to represent. Figure 12–1 features samples of excellent, professionally prepared pieces of literature that promote rehabilitation programs and instructional aids for patients. Keep in mind that undertaking projects of this size may not be considered financially viable until the program is well underway. Of course, the entrepreneurial administrator of the program may investigate the feasibility of obtaining funding from pharmaceutical companies, lung associations, federal grants, or other such sources. (Chapter 15 lists various literature and other sources.)

Initially, the main source of referrals may come from the medical direc-

TABLE 12–2.—EXAMPLE OF ANNOUNCEMENT TO MARKET A PULMONARY
REHABILITATION PROGRAM

Dear Doctor:

Did you know that we are currently doing bedside pulmonary rehabilitation at Grandview?

This new concept, incepted March 1981, is part of a total pulmonary reconditioning program entitled Phase I-IV. Phase I is the actual bedside breathing exercises we can teach your patient. This includes ventilator patients and is considered a part of their weaning process.

Phase II is the ongoing Pulmonary Education classes that we've been doing at Grandview since August 1980. You can refer any patient to this phase: it's free of charge to the patient.

Phase III is the posthospitalization care the patient receives at Southview Hospital's Family Health Center.* Phase III involves the patient having 2-3 visits/week at the Family Health Center for a period of 4-6 weeks. You are sent biweekly reports detailing your patient's progress.

Phase IV is the ongoing care the patient receives after he completes the Phase III portion at the Family Health Center. Phase IV simply means that we continue to see the chronic patient at monthly or bimonthly intervals to reinforce and augment the breathing exercises the patient has already learned.

All patients are seen by qualified pulmonary rehabilitation specialists who receive continual postgraduate training.

In order to have your patient get started on Phase I-IV Pulmonary Rehabilitation, simply write "Phase I-IV Pulmonary Rehab" on your chart orders.

Finally, if you desire a copy of an article on the basics of pulmonary rehabilitation, call me at Grandview, and I'll make sure you receive a copy. Thank you.

Respectfully,

Donald G. Burns, D.O., F.A.C.O.I.,
F.C.C.P.
Medical Director, Respiratory Therapy

*Southview Hospital and Family Health Center (formerly the Ambulatory Care Center) is a freestanding hospital and outpatient facility owned and operated by Grandview Hospital, Dayton, Ohio.

tor of the respiratory therapy department. Secondary sources include other pulmonary physicians, internists, medical residents, rotating interns, and cardiothoracic surgeons. Surprisingly, only a small number of referrals may come from general practitioners due to the simple fact that the family physician may already be referring his chronic obstructive lung disease (COLD) patients to specialists. However, this potential referral source should not be overlooked, because the generalist may consider treating the less severe COLD patient, especially once he is aware that there is a whole group of allied health pulmonary specialists there to assist him.

If a member of the pulmonary rehabilitation department or other staff workers are aware of a patient who may receive benefit by being referred to the program, they should let the pulmonary rehabilitation coordinator know this. The coordinator can then tactfully inquire of the patient's physician whether he would consider allowing the coordinator to perform a

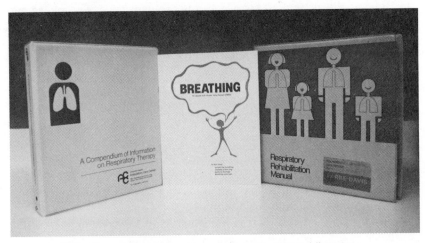

Fig 12–1.—Examples of marketing/educational literature.

preliminary investigation into the possible merits of the patient receiving pulmonary rehabilitation.

The Multidisciplinary Approach

No longer just a buzzword or theoretical concept, the multidisciplinary approach is often the basis for the success of many patient care endeavors, pulmonary rehabilitation notwithstanding. Those institutions without the full command of an eclectic discipline of allied health professionals and ancillary assistants can do just as well, however. They will merely need to shift some of the responsibilities to team members whose skills most nearly match the crucial missing skill. For example, the physical therapist may be able to substitute for the occupational therapist. When the program gets to be of an appreciably large size, and requiring more and more use of a still unavailable discipline, alternatives such as using part-time, pool personnel or even subcontracting are plausible.

The multidisciplinary rehabilitation team would include the following professional representatives: (1) physician, (2) respiratory therapist, (3) registered nurse, (4) physical therapist, (5) occupational therapist, (6) dietician, (7) social worker, (8) pastoral care member, and (9) psychiatrist or psychologist.

It is important to reiterate that this list represents an ideal state. The overall objective of the pulmonary rehabilitation team is to provide a comprehensive, coordinated treatment program for the patient with a chronic lung disease. This objective is met by aiming for these goals:

1. Helping the patient to cope with his problem on a physiologic and psychological level.

2. Assuring that the patient can maintain or even improve his quality of life in the domestic and occupational setting.

3. Allowing the patient to function as much as possible within his home setting with the help of family members as required.

These goals are made possible by having the team help the patient to meet the following *patient-centered* behavioral objectives, with family participation as necessary:

Physician's Role

1. Relates pertinent history, including family history, past illnesses, occupational history, and smoking history.

2. Allows a complete physical examination to be performed.

3. Receives diagnostic tests as determined necessary.

4. Receives all therapy ordered for treatment and relief of symptoms.

5. Seeks information about the disease process of COLD, the prognosis, treatment, and other pertinent information.

6. Seeks treatment at the first sign of impending infection, such as a change in sputum color, amount, or consistency, or for increasing dyspnea or other symptoms of exacerbation of COLD.

Respiratory Therapist's Role

1. Receives all therapy and diagnostic tests provided by the respiratory therapy department as ordered by the physician.

2. Identifies the purpose and basic principles of oxygen therapy, including the associated hazards and benefits.

3. Identifies the purpose, benefit, and basic principles involved in carrying out a breathing treatment.

4. Demonstrates proper operation and maintenance of his breathing machine and/or oxygen equipment.

5. Demonstrates proper cleaning procedure for breathing equipment with a specific attitude of appreciation of why this is so important.

6. Demonstrates knowledge and ability to safely prepare and use medications as part of his breathing treatment.

7. Performs pulmonary hygiene measures safely and effectively with ability to state their purpose and value.

8. Performs the specific routine of postural drainage correctly and safely as directed.

9. Identifies adequate daily fluid intake as also being important to thin and mobilize secretions.

10. Observes sputum characteristics with consideration of the significance of change in color, consistency, or amount.

Registered Nurse's Role

1. Meets basic needs and maintains activities of daily living with necessary nursing assistance.

2. Participates in a coordinated, patient-centered program of daily living activities, therapy, and education.

3. Has status monitored and becomes able to evaluate own status and abilities.

4. Practices all learned techniques and exercises in carrying out activities of daily living on the nursing division.

5. Develops ability to emotionally and psychologically cope with symptoms, the presence of lung disease, and the associated individual implications.

6. Describes in simple terms key structures of the breathing system, the normal breathing process and its importance, and the patient's problem as it hampers breathing.

7. Identifies factors related to the cause of lung disease with an expressed willingness to avoid or control them as part of a prevention and treatment program.

8. Verbalizes names, expected actions, and dosage of medications patient will take at home, as well as how to take them (observations and precautions).

9. Plans for self-care needs at home with input of nursing viewpoint.

Physical Therapist's Role

1. Demonstrates effective breathing within his/her own breathing pattern.

2. Demonstrates ability to control dyspnea by use of learned breathing techniques.

3. Utilizes an effective method to produce a cough.

4. Applies learned relaxation techniques.

5. Applies pacing/phasing techniques in patient's activity.

6. Demonstrates increased tolerance to physical activity.

Occupational Therapist's Role

1. Applies pacing/phasing techniques in patient's daily living skills of activities of daily living, homemaking, work activities, etc.

2. Demonstrates functional level of work tolerance.

3. Achieves improvement in dyspnea classification level at time of discharge.

4. Demonstrates appropriate behavior in seeking or returning to vocational/avocational activities.

5. Maintains level of function appropriate with individual treatment goals.

Dietician's Role

1. Verbalizes key aspects of good basic nutrition.

2. Identifies patient's problems related to nutrition.

3. Verbalizes ways he/she intends to correct nutritional problems.

4. Lists mucus-forming foods.

5. Lists gas-forming and hard-to-digest foods.

6. Demonstrates ability to plan for six feedings each day by writing a week's menus.

7. Verbalizes the role of fluid intake in relation to mucus production.

8. Demonstrates the ability to identify high potassium foods if needed because of medications.

Social Worker's Role

1. Demonstrates in discussion and planning a realistic view of patient's illness and its implications for lifestyle and the family unit.

2. Verbalizes plans for any necessary lifestyle modifications that will encourage patient's well-being and optimal functioning.

3. Demonstrates understanding of the emotional impact of the illness on all family members, with ability to handle feelings and alter patterns of interaction to lessen emotional strain and maintain the family unit.

4. Aware of and utilizes as needed the counseling, referral, and discharge-planning services offered by the social service department.

5. Aware of and utilizes as necessary community resources to assist in meeting financial, vocational, social, counseling and health service needs.

Pastoral Care Role

1. Identifies the availability of pastoral care services to patient and family as desired while hospitalized.

2. Gives sacraments as desired and appropriate (Catholic patients).

3. Gives the patient opportunity to express anxieties and concerns, discuss problems and solutions, and receive supportive pastoral counseling and guidance.

4. Copes with the experience of respiratory illness with all the implications of symptoms, hospitalization, necessary therapy, and rehabilitation measures with the opportunity for spiritual, emotional, and psychological support.

5. Identifies how and when pastoral care services can be obtained as needed and desired after discharge.

Psychiatrist's or Psychologist's Role

1. Allows patient to verbalize doubts, fears, and anxieties related to the changes in lifestyle and relationships which occur in the presence of lung disease.

2. Helps patient learn to accept the diagnosis and therefore the treatment for COLD.

3. Develops the ability to cope with psychological defense mechanisms such as denial, regression, and suppression.*

Obtaining Personnel

Pulmonary rehabilitation personnel are made, not born. If we pick one particular key member of the rehabilitation team, the respiratory therapist for example, we would see that he or she represents a typical respiratory school graduate therapist who through a certain number of years of working in respiratory therapy now finds himself working more and more exclusively with convalescing COLD patients. He may find that he has much interest in working one-on-one with the same patient for days or weeks and derives immense satisfaction in whatever salvaging of the patient's pulmonary reserve he can bring about. The personality profile and job-type characteristics of the potential pulmonary rehab worker would ideally include that he (1) likes the educational factor of dealing with COLD patients, (2) has a lot of patience and is not easily frustrated, (3) is able to work alongside other health professionals and share responsibilities, successes, and failures, (4) possesses classic traits of a team worker, (5) understands and willingly accepts the fact that because of the newness of pulmonary rehabilitation the techniques used in the field are not of a cookbook methodology, and (6) has entrepreneurial ability.

The above listed virtues more or less profile the desired attributes of any member of the pulmonary rehabilitation team. While we all like to think of ourselves as pioneers and capable of innovation, we often do not get the opportunity to demonstrate these attributes if indeed they do exist (which they may not for all of us). Those involved with the rehabilitation of COLD patients must possess these attributes: they will have many opportunities to practice them.

Where will your pulmonary rehabilitation personnel be recruited? Some

---

*Information on professional roles, with the exception of physician's and psychiatrist/psychologist's roles, from St. John Hospital Respiratory Program, Cleveland. Used by permission.

areas of current or past work experience by a therapist or nurse may lend itself naturally to the practice of pulmonary rehabilitation. One example may be the therapist or nurse who has worked on a postventilator unit, where daily experiences of working with convalescing patients are similar to many of the restorative procedures used in pulmonary rehabilitation. Therapists and nurses with a flair for teaching and who possess the necessary close communication skills needed for long-term patient care are good candidates.

Once the decision to start a pulmonary rehabilitation program is made, a full commitment must be made to ensure that the required personnel will be available to operate the program. The key personnel functioning in the program will be the respiratory therapist and nurse. Whether or not they work in the program full- or part-time is inversely related to the number of new patients being referred and old patients being treated. It would certainly not be presumptuous to say that once the program gets underway, the transition from part- to full-time will be a direct result of (1) more initial referrals being entered into the program, requiring more work-up time on these patients, and (2) as a result of this, there will be more and more patients scattered throughout all phases of the program.

The other members of the team—physical and occupation therapists, dietary, social workers, etc.—may not be required on a full-time basis, but will perform their function initially and periodically as required by each individual patient's needs.

One final word on the subject is that a sense of permanency and readiness to serve on the part of the rehabilitation team must be perceived by the physicians referring their patients to the program. All the best publicity and marketing attempts will not maintain a program if it lacks continuity, substance, and a sense of presence.

Where and When is Pulmonary Rehabilitation Performed?

Logistically, pulmonary rehabilitative procedures are performed in four areas: (1) *inpatient*, at the bedside; (2) *inpatient*, in the pulmonary rehabilitation clinic; (3) *outpatient*, where patient has regular appointment at specific intervals; and (4) *home care*, performed in patient's residence or nursing home.

The first three situations allow the full use of most equipment or supplies that might be needed. The last, home care, will be discussed in Chapter 13. Other than some limitation of equipment uses at the bedside (e.g., treadmill), the main difference of the bedside vs. the outpatient or home-care situation will be the status of the patient at the time. Obviously, patients who have just been weaned from the ventilator and are still very weak will be treated at the bedside. Conversely, ambulating or even semiambulating patients can be treated in the department clinic, where a greater access of equipment is available.

Phase I-IV Concept

The concept of Phase I-IV was developed at Southview Hospital and Family Health Center in Dayton, Ohio, in order to (1) simplify and allow a more sequential approach to the patient's pulmonary rehabilitative needs at any given point and (2) provide a comprehensive plan of care that takes into consideration the continuing care the patient will need because of the very chronicity of his disease.

In brief, the Phase I-IV concept is a logical categorization of the whole pulmonary rehabilitative process that informs the physician and other interested parties (e.g., third-party payers) approximately where the patient is in this process. This categorization also allows the physician and other interested parties to have a general idea of where the patient is at prognostically, relative to his disease state (see Table 12–2).

Here is a synopsis of how the Phase I-IV concept works (in this description, the patient is assumed to be an inpatient): *Phase I* is the initial bedside breathing training and low-level exercises taught to the patient. *Phase II* is the ongoing pulmonary education process, both formal and informal, that the patient receives. *Phase III* is the posthospitalization or outpatient care the patient receives. This involves having the patient visit two to three times per week for 4 to 6 weeks. *Phase IV* refers to the regular follow-up visits at spaced intervals, relative to the patient's condition and needs. Usually this will mean that the patient is seen at monthly or bimonthly intervals and then on a quarterly, semiannual, or even annual basis.

Another way to view the Phase I-IV concept is to see this as the vehicle that initiates the rehabilitative process. The ordering physician simply writes, "Start pulmonary rehab, Phase I-IV" on the patient's chart. Once the pulmonary rehabilitation order has been written, it is imperative that a senior member of the rehabilitation team (in the author's hospital, this is the respiratory therapist who also serves as the pulmonary rehabilitation coordinator) expediently perform the initial assessment of the patient and report this to the physician. Again, it is important to remember that expediency is crucial to the success of a newly created pulmonary rehabilitation program.

Charting and Reporting Systems

Charting takes on a different aspect for the therapist who is used to charting "Med neb with Bronkosol 0.5 cc, 10 minutes, NC, P:82–96. Sm. SOB" (translated: Medication nebulizer with Bronkosol 0.5 cc for 10 minutes. No cough. Pulse rate 82 at beginning of treatment, 96 at end of treatment. Some shortness of breath.). Charting rehabilitative notes of any kind necessitates not only spelling out (literally and figuratively) what has been done, but also including anecdotal information. It is this author's strong opinion that full and regularly occurring documentation of the patient's progress is mandatory. Other than the obvious reason that a chart, or any medical report for that matter, is a legal document, there are other equally good reasons: (1) For the program just starting, thorough and professional documentation gives an opportunity to show the seriousness and the intended depth of the program. (2) For insurance and medical disability cases, proper and professional documentation is mandatory. (3) Documentation can provide statistical information for medical and psychosocial research.

The argument is often heard that, "Doctors (or others) just don't like to read lengthy reports." If they do not, then that is all the more reason to document progress and events, because it is when something goes wrong with the patient that full validation of the patient's care is desirable.

There should not be an overwhelming array of paperwork generated in spite of the caveat to chart promptly and fully. Inpatient documentation will occur on the patient's chart, although a separate page should be reserved for this rather than charting on the standard IPPB/Aerosol/CPT form. There are three good reasons for this: (1) There is an uninterrupted chronology of the patient's rehabilitative events readily available. (2) The separate sheet again serves as a psychological and marketing tool, reminding all concerned parties of the depth and breadth of the program. (3) It provides additional impetus, clarity of objectives being met, and easily perused validation for insurance companies dubious of the benefits of pulmonary rehabilitation. Tables 12–3 to 12–5 and Figure 12–2 illustrate the types of report systems used at the author's institution. Take special note of Tables 12–5 and 12–6, which typify a comprehensive report sent to a physician after he has referred a patient directly to the outpatient portion of the program. One final note is that proper grammatical syntax, spelling, and punctuation are essential.

Equipment*

Equipment can be separated into two categories: (1) the equipment used for testing and evaluating the extent of pulmonary disability, and (2) the equipment used for actual rehabilitative procedures.

---

*The references to or illustration of any equipment in this chapter (or in other chapters) do not constitute any endorsement or testimonial of the equipment. At the current time and pursuant to our program's goal, the equipment we use for the most part fulfills our needs. Both authors, J. A. O'Ryan and D. G. Burns, are available for consultation in the matter of equipment purchases.

TABLE 12–3.—EXAMPLE OF INPATIENT INITIAL ASSESSMENT REPORT

The following is the initial pulmonary rehabilitation evaluation done on Betty Smith. It was performed on May 27, 1982, per Dr. Jones' order. Mrs. Smith was admitted to Grandview Hospital on May 25, 1982, with the chief complaint of severe dyspnea secondary to COLD. She was seen by Dr. Jones, whose impression was that she had emphysema, chronic bronchitis, and probable early cor pulmonale. Her pulmonary function reveals severe obstructive pulmonary mechanics possibly associated with restrictive lung disease.

Mrs. Smith presents as a 49-year-old female in no respiratory distress at rest. She has smoked one to three packs of cigarettes per day for 20 years, but quit on admission to Grandview Hospital. She has experienced shortness of breath for 2 years, and it seemed to increase 1 year ago. She has a cough productive of thick pink-to-white sputum, especially in the morning and at night. She states that any exertion such as vacuuming, bed making, or carrying out the trash causes severe dyspnea. Mrs. Smith's son is living with her at this time, and he does help with work around the house. Mrs. Smith relates that she does not eat properly. She would like to be able to ride her bicycle, walk around the block, and clean her own house. I believe Mrs. Smith could benefit from the following pulmonary rehabilitation program:
   1. Patient education concerning her lung disease.
   2. Diaphragmatic pursed-lip breathing techniques.
   3. Biofeedback with relaxation techniques.
   4. Psychological support to maintain her nonsmoking status.
   5. Consultation with a dietician regarding the patient's poor nutrition.
   6. Outpatient therapy following discharge from Grandview Hospital.
Thank you for this referral.

Signed

Equipment costs involved with starting a pulmonary rehabilitation program should be inherently minimal. Basically, the pulmonary function equipment currently used to test other patients is also used for the rehabilitation patients. A separate filing system should be instituted for the purposes of allowing quick access and for future research projects.

Possibly the only capital equipment expenditures that could not enjoy a dual use would be those pieces limited to rehabilitative measures only, e.g., full-length mirror, portable stairs, and stationary bicycle. All other items can be used by nonpulmonary rehabilitation patients as long as there does not exist the possibility of double-booking of the same piece of equipment. Optimally and optimistically, however, a separate area with equipment dedicated to rehabilitation patients only should be the ultimate goal.

Table 12–6 lists the testing and rehabilitative equipment required. For those departments with small budgets allocated for these types of purchases, funding from local or state lung associations, industy or federal grants are possibilities.

Departmental Layout

The ideal rehabilitation department will be described, although many institutions may not be able (or willing) to commit such a large capital and

SOUTHVIEW HOSPITAL AND
FAMILY HEALTH CENTER
PULMONARY REHABILITATION DEPT.

ORDER:

DIAGNOSIS (and comments):

PATIENT:

DATE	TIME	RANGE OF MOTION	EXERCISE	EDUCATION	THERAPY	MISC.	MISC. THERP.
		a. DBE d. Elbow-to-Elbow g. Lateral Bending b. Kneebends e. Arm-Shoulder h. Modified push-ups c. Chairbends Girdle i. others: f. Waistbends	Treadmill Bicycle Walking	Films Tapes A & P	Med Neb IS HA ABG CPT PPD		

Fig 12-2.—Example of a departmental charting form.

TABLE 12–4.—EXAMPLE OF OUTPATIENT INITIAL ASSESSMENT REPORT

Dear Dr._____:

The following report concerns the pulmonary assessment done on William Blake on March 31, 1983.

Mr. Blake presents as a thin, elderly male who appears to be somewhat short of breath at rest. He presently uses home oxygen at 3 L 1 min. No cyanosis was noted.

Mr. Blake states he rarely coughs; this only occurs during chest colds. He does have exertional dyspnea, which has worsened during the past 2 years. Mr. Blake related that he smoked for 50 years, but quit 2 years ago. He stated that he would like to be able to care for himself and his house sufficiently to be able to live at home again.

The results of Mr. Blake's chest examination follow:

1. Breath sounds were clear, but diminished on auscultation.
2. Movement of the chest cage was equal bilaterally, both anteriorly and posteriorly.
3. Movement of the diaphragm was fair, with excessive use of the accessory muscles for ventilation noted.
4. No scars or other markings were observed on the chest.

Because Mr. Blake had a chest x-ray during his recent hospitalization, this will not be repeated. A sputogenesis was done, and the results should be available by the end of this week. Because Mr. Blake has not had a pulmonary function test since 1977, this will be done next week. He will also have a cardiopulmonary stress test in the near future.

Mr. Blake will be receiving therapy two to three times per week for the next 6 weeks. I have outlined the following program for him:

1. Diaphragmatic breathing retraining.
2. Range of motion and chest mobilization exercises.
3. Coordination of walking and other activities with breathing.
4. Relaxation techniques, using biofeedback.
5. Treadmill exercise to increase the patient's exercise tolerance.

Progress reports will be done biweekly, and Mr. Blake will be reassessed in 6 weeks. If you have any questions, comments, or suggestions, please call me at 435-6500, ext. 313.

Signed

floorspace expenditure to such a venture (and rightfully so, since it would be prudent to expand only as the need exists).

Many current successful pulmonary rehabilitation facilities are merely shared space with other outpatient treatment areas or are former office or storage spaces converted for rehabilitative use. Many of the basic treatment modalities used in pulmonary rehabilitation are borrowed directly from current respiratory and chest physical modalities practiced in the inpatient setting. This means that storage of disposables should not pose a problem, because most of the items, e.g., aerosol units and cannulae, can be stored with inpatient items of the same type.

Those involved with planning of the rehabilitation area should also give consideration to dual use of the facility for conventional outpatient therapy, i.e., the nonrehabilitative patient such as the acute bronchitis or pneumonia patient. In fact, it does not hurt to market this aspect of your facility, because the dual-use benefit should please physicians in light of its conve-

TABLE 12–5.—Example of Outpatient Reassessment Report

Dear Dr._____:

The following report is a pulmonary reassessment on William Blake, who has been receiving pulmonary reconditioning twice a week. Mr. Blake's visits were reduced earlier this month when he moved back to his own home.

Mr. Blake has appeared to do well in his pulmonary reconditioning program, as evidenced by his successful return to living in his own home. He practices diaphragmatic breathing and does the range of motion and chest mobilization exercises at least twice daily and uses diaphragmatic breathing techniques to accomplish his activities of daily living. Mr. Blake has learned to cope more successfully with his dyspnea using these techniques. He is able to walk for longer distances and has been encouraged to walk for additional exercise at home, which should increase his exercise tolerance. Mr. Blake has also been taught relaxation techniques, because he has a tendency toward being tense that increases his problem with dyspnea.

On April 27, an arterial blood gas was drawn after Mr. Blake was *off* O_2 for 30 minutes. The results were as follows: pH 7.40; P_{CO_2} 34.1; P_{O_2} 47.1; BE -3; HCO_3 19.2; $CO_{2_{ct}}$ 20.2; HbO_2 82.2%.

Dr. Jones was notified of these results and ordered that Mr. Blake remain on continuous O_2 at 3 L/min. Mr. Blake seems to be having difficulty accepting the reality of wearing oxygen 24 hours a day. I have talked with him at length concerning this problem, but his acceptance continues to be minimal. Mr. Blake has stated that if he had to be on O_2 for the rest of his life, he "might as well be at the end of a rope." He has made other overt references to his impending death, and I have discussed this with Janet Cowan, R.N., our geriatric nurse practitioner. She felt during a previous tandem counseling session that Mr. Blake may commit suicide and that his target date is the end of the summer. He has stated several times that he must make a decision of some type by then, because he feels he can't live alone during the winter, but he doesn't want to move back with his niece. In talking with him, I feel he is not leaving himself many options.

On a more positive note, Mr. Blake has considered marrying a woman with whom he is friends and has not closed the door on this possibility. It would be possible for a psychiatric social worker from the Senior Citizen's Center to visit Mr. Blake to help him work out some of his problems. I will keep you informed of Mr. Blake's progress, as he will continue therapy twice a week for the next 4 weeks. Please call me at 435-6500, ext. 313, if you have any questions, comments, or suggestions.

Signed

nience to their non-COLD patients. It should also please cost-benefit conscientious administrations. (Again, entrepreneurship cannot be overstressed!)

Figure 12–3 depicts an ideal layout for a pulmonary rehabilitation room. This layout automatically serves the nonchronic short-term (e.g., pneumonia) pulmonary patient, also.

Summary

Physical size of a pulmonary rehabilitation department can vary from a converted storage closet to one that is several hundred or thousands of square feet. The medical director of the program, the technical director, and pulmonary rehabilitation coordinator must work in a cooperative spirit with the administrators to assess the amount of area needed.

TABLE 12–6.—Testing and Rehabilitation Equipment Used in Pulmonary Rehabilitation

Testing Equipment

1. Pulmonary function unit–capable of spirometry, lung volumes and diffusion studies.
2. Cardiopulmonary stress testing devices–capable of full O_2 and CO_2 ventilatory measurements.
3. Arterial blood gas analyzer–to measure baseline, with and without O_2 use studies and postexercise O_2 levels.
4. Ear oximeter–to measure O_2 desaturation during exercise.

Rehabilitation Equipment

1. Treadmill–for cardiopulmonary stress testing and exercise training.
2. Stationary bicycle–as an augmentative and/or substitute exercising device (see Chapter 6 on treadmill vs. bicycling).
3. Full-length Mirror–to teach proper breathing stance.
4. Tilt-table–for cardiopulmonary therapy and to teach supine diaphragmatic breathing.
5. Portable steps–to teach breath conservation while stair climbing.
6. Sandbags–to teach diaphragmatic breathing.
7. Miscellaneous respiratory therapy equipment–aerosol-producing units, incentive spirometry, IPPB machine, inspiratory muscle training devices.

Likewise, staffing will depend on the size of the program and number of patients to be treated. Where will referred patients come from? Through your marketing efforts, will you in time be getting almost as many patients from the general practitioner as you are from the specialist?

For any reader who may even be the least bit stifled by the thought of

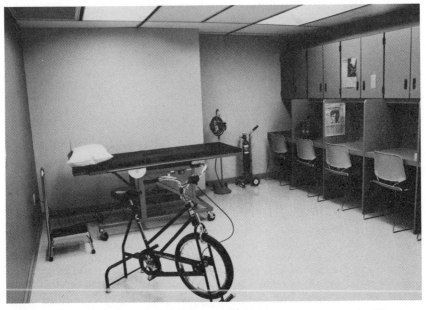

Fig 12–3.—Example of a pulmonary rehabilitation treatment room. (Courtesy of Southview Hospital and Family Health Center, Dayton, Ohio.)

TABLE 12-7.—HOW TO START A REHABILITATION PROGRAM

1. If you want and need a rehab program for your patients with COPD–have one!
2. Don't wait until you have the money!
3. The key to a successful pulmonary rehab program is a method designed to teach the patient and family to live with emphysema and chronic bronchitis.
4. The most important part of a rehab program is *one* interested person. One person must be appointed and be called the Rehab Therapist or Rehab Nurse. Why not use one of your respiratory therapy positions for this? It might require some reorganization and reassessment, but it can often be done without significant additional expense.
5. The second important part is a system to get the patient in the program, to teach the patient, to follow up the patient, and to recover expenses.
6. Set up a corner in the therapy department or somewhere on the medical floor that can be used parttime by the rehab person for patient teaching.
7. You need visual aids, but why not a picture book you make yourself? Get the CIBA^R COPD and Asthma books and cut out needed pictures. Take your own pictures of therapy with a Kodak^R instamatic. Ask your drug detail men for free booklets. There is a gold mine of goodies available.
8. Talk your volunteers (i.e., hospital auxiliary) into a donation of several dollars for printed home aids.
9. Write up a protocol of what you are going to teach or do. Have guidelines for stop points if you want to exercise patients. Talk to a sympathetic physician; get him to back your ideas. If he doesn't want to get involved, forget the exercise part and get started with the patient teaching. The rest will follow.
10. Start with one patient. If you find it is more economical to do your program in groups, add that to your system. Word about your good work will spread. Don't try to take care of the whole state or whole country. Take care of your patients at your hospital. You can always grow bigger and better once you get it off the ground.
11. Talk with your financial manager in the business office. Establish a reasonable charge for your service. Ask your finance officer to set up a meeting with your insurance carriers so they will pay for this important service. You have to say it in their language, or it will be turned down.
12. Good Luck!

(From Petty T.: Pulmonary rehabilitation. *Continuing Education* 9:36, 1978. Used by permission.)

undertaking the task of starting a pulmonary rehabilitation program, 12 very pragmatic tips from Thomas L. Petty, M.D., are offered (see Table 12–7).

Suggested Reading

1. MacDonell R.J.: The pulmonary rehabilitation maze. *Respir. Care* 28:180, 1983.
2. May D.F., Kenny W.R.: Pulmonary rehabilitation: Dealing effectively with chronic pulmonary disease. *J. Med. Assoc. Ga.* 69:205, 1980.
3. O'Ryan J.A.: Blue Cross respiratory project. January 1979 (unpublished data).
4. O'Ryan, J.A., : *Compendium of Information on Respiratory Therapy at Grandview Hospital's Ambulatory Care Center* (notebook). Available from author (Route 725, Centerville, OH 45459.)
5. White B., Andrews J.L., et al.: Pulmonary rehabilitation in an ambulatory group practice setting. *Med. Clin. North Am.* 63:379, 1979.

13 / Home Care

JERRY A. O'RYAN, B.S., R.R.T.

HOME CARE is a natural and logical extension of the patient's in-hospital pulmonary rehabilitation program. The multidisciplinary approach discussed in Chapter 12 still applies when instituting home care, although the depth and extent of involvement of most members of the pulmonary rehabilitation team will be minimized as far as on-site activities are concerned. The two members of the team whose skills will be required on a more regular basis in the home are the respiratory therapist and nurse.

This chapter will discuss the role of the home-care team, especially the respiratory therapist and nurse. It will also detail the responsibilities the patient and his family will play in home care. Equipment used in the home will be discussed along with the safety measures to be taken when using medical equipment in the home setting. Finally, the costs of home care and the problems that accompany these costs will be discussed.

The Role of the Home-Care Team

On an in-depth basis, the respiratory therapist and nurse assume the larger roles in the patient's home care. This is because their duties inherently focus more on the specific (i.e., medical) needs of the patient in his home. The respiratory therapist will tend to the patient's bronchopulmonary needs, while the nurse will focus on other bodily systems requiring skilled nursing care on an interval basis.

If the other members of the pulmonary rehabilitation team have performed their functions well prior to the patient's discharge, then they will have few posthospital obligations, usually only occasional home visits or consulting over the phone. Table 13–1 lists some of the duties the members of the team may find necessary to perform as part of the patient's predischarge planning. (The reader may also wish to refer to Chapter 12 for a review of each team member's general function.) We will now return to the home-care duties of the respiratory therapist and nurse, who, as time goes by, may find their duties possibly expanding and becoming more eclectic in scope and practice as they perform many of the functions of their fellow team members. Table 13–2 lists the general functions that the respiratory therapist and nurse perform in the home-care setting.

199

TABLE 13–1.—DISCHARGE PLANNING DUTIES OF PULMONARY
REHABILITATION TEAM

TEAM MEMBER	DUTIES
Physician	Does final assessment of patient, writes all drug and equipment prescriptions.
Respiratory therapist	Evaluates all facets of patient's respiratory status, reviews equipment, and supplies needs.
Nurse	Assesses all bodily needs, singularly and as a whole, and writes initial home-care plan.
Physical therapist	Evaluates patient's current musculoskeletal status, reviews all self-care patient must perform with self and family.
Dietician	Writes home nutrition plan, makes sure patient will have adequate nutritive intake or makes alternate plans (e.g., Meals on Wheels).
Occupational therapist	Reassesses patient's gains since occupational therapy began in-hospital and informs home-care team of strengths and weaknesses.
Psychiatrist/psychologist	Writes patient profile summary and shares *allowable* areas with home-care team.
Social worker	Checks and double checks to make certain all outside agencies involved with patient's home care are ready to assist and have all red tape out of way.
Pastoral member	Makes arrangements to see patient on regular basis once patient is home or sees as needed.

The first few visits should give the home-care team a good overview of conditions in the home, the patient's coping and compliance abilities, and how the patient and family interact with each other. Each visit allows an excellent opportunity for reinforcement of prior hospital learning. Ongoing evaluations of the patient and family's learning domains, i.e., cognitive, affective, and psychomotor, can be assessed where they relate to care of the patient.

TABLE 13–2.—HOME-CARE FUNCTIONS OF RESPIRATORY THERAPIST AND NURSE

Respiratory Therapist
1. Assess general pulmonary status and reeducate patient in deficient areas.
2. Evaluate and monitor equipment use, care, and provide correction and reinforcement of any deficient areas.
3. Review pulmonary rehabilitation breathing training and exercises taught in hospital.
4. Write summary of visit and send to physician.*
Nurse
1. Assess general bodily status as a whole and singularly, noting areas requiring greater self-care or medical attention by physician.
2. Review all medications and ascertain if patient is being compliant; correct deficient areas.
3. Perform needed skilled nursing functions that cannot be performed by patient or family, e.g., tracheostomy tube changes, deep-wound dressing changes, etc.
4. Write summary of visit and send to physician.*

*Reports can be summated together.

If there is to be both therapist and nurse visitation, then the two should make the first few visits together if possible. This provides both with an initial common base of comparison for any future communication regarding the patient's progress, compliance, and general status.

How often should the patient be visited? Depending on the continuing severity of his disease and complexity of medical care required, visits may range from daily (initially) to weekly to biweekly or monthly. If more closely intervaled visits are needed, then consideration will need to be given to using a private home health agency. (A later section in this chapter discusses home-care costs and alternatives to hospital-based personnel performing closely intervaled visits.) Home-care visitations are not to supplant the patient and family's responsibilities of home care. Instead, home visits are meant to provide an ongoing monitoring and appraisal of the patient's health status and to reinforce all prior learning.

A written report of each visit should be made and entered into the patient's standing outpatient file in the home-care or rehabilitation clinic. A copy is to be mailed to the physician. The report should include all the following data and observations as they pertain to the patient:

1. Date, time, and length of visit.

2. Condition of patient and immediate living area prior to rendering any actual care or other intervention.

3. Details of care or other activities performed.

4. Any unusual changes in bodily functions since last visit (e.g., stool, urine, sputum, vital signs).

5. Notation of any areas of deficiency requiring correction.

6. Notation of any new advice, instructions given, or changes made.

7. Anecdotal remarks denoting any changes in psychosocial profile, economic status, etc.

8. State clearly any suggested changes in therapy modalities, medication dosages, frequency change of visits, etc.

Table 13–3 is an example of a home-care visit report as performed by a private home-care consulting group. A hospital-based team would write essentially the same report.

The Patient and Family's Responsibilities

The patient and his family must be prepared for his home care well in advance of the patient's dismissal from the hospital. This can be done with confidence and ease in the patient whose condition is stable and who has a good prognosis for eventual home care. A family conference with the core group of relatives or friends participating in the patient's home care is the first step. It is here that certain individuals can be singled out as being the more responsible members of the family.

TABLE 13–3.—SAMPLE OF HOME-CARE VISIT REPORT (INITIAL VISIT)*

Patient: J.W.	Medications: Lanoxin 0.25 mg QD
Diagnosis: COLD, CHF	Lasix 40 mgs QD
Physician: Dr. R. Leffler	Alupent 0.3cc
Hospital Source: Miami Valley	Vital Signs: B/P 140/90
Mentation: Very good	Pulse 82

This report details the results of a home-care visit on your patient, Mr. J.W.

Mr. W. has been residing in his home since his hospital discharge on 8/10. Residing with him are his wife and teenaged daughter, both of whom take an active part in Mr. W.'s home care.

Mr. W. is on a "Mini-O$_2$" oxygen concentrator at 2 L/min, 18 hours a day minimum. He appears to tolerate the oxygen well and states he has no problem with the device itself as far as cleaning, maintenance, and general operation of the unit. He also takes a medication nebulizer (0.3cc Alupent in a 5.0cc saline diluent) treatment BID for relief of intermittent bronchospasm. This is tolerated well with only moderate coughing and sputum production of a light yellow, semiviscid quality observed after most treatments. This is confirmed by our observation of a treatment during a visit.

Nursing care procedures consist mainly of monitoring vital signs, checking for medication compliance, and answering questions about Mr. W.'s general concerns about his heart. Mr. W. states, "I'm more afraid of my heart than my lungs . . . after all I've lived with this danged breathing problem for years, but this heart dropsy is new to me." He was reassured that his medications would keep his heart in check.

Observations of the patient's home environment reveals a cheerful, well-kept home. Both wife and daughter are there most of the time to assist Mr. W. with his health-care needs. Mr. W. prefers to "do for myself" and expresses this desire at every opportunity, possibly to the chagrin of his wife and daughter, as they show a sincere desire to help him.

Our only concerns were his increased sodium intake habits and his tendency to be a little too self-dependent. We will contact a dietician for the former problem and talk with Mr. W.'s hospital psychologist about the latter situation. We also would like to get your permission to reduce Mr. W.'s bronchodilator treatment to a prn basis only, based on our current assessment of his bronchopulmonary status (auscultation revealed essentially clear lungs prior to his observed medication nebulizer therapy).

Thank you for reading our report. We would welcome any comments, questions, or suggestions regarding our care of your patient.

Signed

*Courtesy of Respiratory Consultants of Dayton, 3490 Upper Bellbrook Rd., Bellbrook, OH 45305.

The patient and family will need to know all aspects of the patient's home-care needs. This can be compartmentalized into two areas: (1) general health care, and (2) equipment operation and maintenance. Table 13–4 lists some of the possible duties these two areas will comprise. Whether the patient or a family member actually performs the function is directly related to the condition and ability of the patient and the fact that some functions may not be of a self-care nature. (The reader is also referred to Chapter 11 for more complete information on the subject of patient and family education.)

TABLE 13–4.—HOME-CARE RESPONSIBILITIES OF PATIENT AND FAMILY

1. Observe as closely as possible all health and safety regulations as directed by pulmonary rehabilitation team.
2. Report the first signs of infections, e.g., change in sputum color, tracheostomy, or other open wound drainage.
3. Maintain a conscientious program of properly cleaning and storing all equipment between uses.
4. Keep a medical diary on a daily or weekly basis that notes subjective feelings regarding progress, feelings about prognosis, etc.
5. Daily perform all phases of breathing training and exercises as prescribed by respiratory therapist.
6. (Family only) Show constructive support to patient and his well-being. Do not patronize or have paternalistic attitude toward patient.
7. Keep all outside home appointments, e.g., physician office visit, outpatient clinic.
8. Learn to be more and more independent of home-care team at a rate and progress that does not put patient's health in jeopardy.

Requirements For Safe Home Care

Assuming that the greater majority of the home-care equipment and supplies will be respiratory in nature, the respiratory therapist will be the main team member responsible for ordering the initial equipment and supplies and teaching its proper use and cleaning for in-home use. Whenever possible, the therapist should arrange for the equipment to be delivered to the hospital at least a few days prior to the patient's discharge to allow the patient and family firsthand experience prior to its use in the home setting. In fact, the home-care equipment should, as far as possible, totally replace similar hospital devices. For example, the patient would now start using his own aerosol, intermittent positive-pressure breathing (IPPB), and even suction machine right at the hospital bedside. Cleaning solutions, usually a vinegar and water mixture, can also be set up by the patient's sink. Return demonstrations on a daily basis are highly recommended.

A cursory visit by the home-care team to the patient's home prior to his discharge is an excellent idea. This affords an opportunity to check out the conduciveness of the patient's place of residence for safe and effective home care. Areas to be carefully scrutinized include the following:

1. Presence of adequate and safe electrical outlets where equipment may be used.

2. General cleanliness of house, notably lack of vermin or rodents, and adequate screening to keep out flies and mosquitos.

3. Hazardous areas in or around the house that may pose a safety problem. Examples are broken steps, drafty windows and doors, faulty furnace (especially if gas or oil), inadequate plumbing.

If the patient is on any critical life support equipment (oxygen concentrator, ventilator, kidney dialysis), then the local life squad must be notified. The utility company also needs to be contacted so that they can promptly restore electrical power in case of an outage, or supply a temporary generator. Some utilities also allow a medical discount for patients using electrically powered life support equipment at home. This will be of special value to the patients on fixed incomes.

Maintaining Therapy Standards in the Home-Care Setting

The home-care patient essentially follows the same regimen he learned while still an inpatient. Modifications and additions can be made as required by a survey of the patient's domestic setting. A simplistic example is the patient who received intensive walking exercise on a treadmill in the hospital and who will now have to transfer that training effect to conventional walking. (See Chapter 6 for details of walking.)

The patient will need to adapt many of the modalities learned in the formal pulmonary rehabilitation program to his particular home setting. Fancy hospital tilt-tables may be replaced with a bed made to slant by propping wood blocks under it. Wood boards, covered with the thickness of a folded blanket and propped at an angle against a bed or other solid stationary object, also make an excellent tilt-table. A modified effect can be gained with pillows placed under the hips.

Pacing of activities must be done if the patient is to perform effective and efficient activities of daily living in the home. Daily breathing and exercise sessions to reinforce previously learned activities and augment the patient's current level of health are mandatory.

There is a curious panacea-type attitude that many patients develop. Another term coined for this is the "hold-over" effect. The patient seems to feel that all the rehabilitative training performed in the hospital or on an intermittent outpatient basis will now, in effect, tide him over for an indefinite period of time. The patient must be made to thoroughly understand that there is no magic "time-release" component to previously performed exercises; all pulmonary rehabilitation modalities must be performed on a regular basis in order to maintain any degree of fitness.

This section could not end without telling the reader the true story of the patient who just could not quite bring herself to stop smoking. She was cutting down on cigarette consumption, fortunately, but for an added therapeutic effect, an antidote if you will, the patient told of this self-prescribed maneuver: "Since I still do smoke a wee bit (four to six cigarettes a day), I ward off all the bad effects of each cigarette by going through the entire regimen of breathing exercises right after I smoke each cigarette."

Selecting Home-Care Equipment

It is the physician's responsibility to write a prescription for each piece of equipment and supply item that will be required for the patient's home-care needs. The respiratory therapist, nurse, and physical therapist can make up the list of items they believe the patient will need. This list is then presented to the physician for approval and prescription writing.

It is highly preferable that all durable medical equipment (DME) be rented until a decision can be made as to what items will actually be needed on a long-term basis. There is also often a tendency to overstock on items; this presents an unnecessary financial burden on patients who must pay a percentage of the amount not covered by insurance.

The required equipment should be obtained from mainly one DME dealer if possible. Needless to say, the dealer chosen should be of the highest integrity and have 24-hour service. Obtaining all or as much equipment as possible from one dealer minimizes the record keeping and phone listings the family will have to keep. This also serves as an impetus to the dealer selected to provide quality, expedient service. Fragmenting the equipment order to a multitude of dealers out of a misguided sense of equality has no place in home care. (The duties of the DME dealer are detailed in Chapter 8 under the discussion of Oxygen Delivery Systems.)

The actual equipment and ancillary items a patient will require are based on his individual needs. For example, a COLD patient requiring continuous oxygen only will need only an oxygen concentrator and appropriate tubing, humidifiers, and backup system. A COLD patient with a permanent tracheostomy will require additional items such as suction apparatus, tracheostomy-cleaning trays and solutions, dressing changes, etc.

It is not the intention of this chapter to list each and every piece of home-care equipment and supply item available. Such a list could never be complete nor up to date. However, it is important to know what are the desirable characteristics of good home-care equipment. Home-care equipment may not be of hospital grade, per se, but it must be able to tolerate the daily wear and tear of an individual's use of it. Home-care equipment for the most part must meet many of the same Underwriter's Laboratories (UL) and FDA criteria that hospital-grade equipment does. In fact, home-care equipment should not only meet but exceed hospital standards, because it may often be used in less than desirable, i.e., nonsupervised, situations in the home environment. Table 13–5 suggests some of the physical and operating characteristics of home-care equipment.

Assessing the Quality of Home Care

By continual assessment of the quality of home care, it is hoped that such close scrutiny of the patient's physiologic and psychological responses to his care and experiences in the home setting will reflect a "standard of care equal to a level acceptable in the hospital setting." *That is what defines quality home care.* To illustrate this standard in an analogy, one only has to be reminded of the classic scale used to grade good nursing home

TABLE 13–5.—DESIRED OPERATING CHARACTERISTICS
OF HOME-CARE EQUIPMENT

CHARACTERISTIC	DESIRED ATTRIBUTES
Shape and size	Small, square, furniture-like design (e.g., concentrator), on wheels or casters if needs to be moved periodically; aesthetically pleasing.
Safety features	UL, FDA approved; fail-safe alarms; battery backup if possible; color coding of tubes, manifolds to prevent inadvertent mistakes when reconnecting.
Ease of operation	Dials, levers, knobs and other controls are large enough to grasp and turn, twist, push or pull, requires no complicated, ambidextrous movements; controls should be in logical sequence.
Sensibility	Takes into account senile or pathologic deficiencies of hearing or seeing; alarms or other audiosensors are comfortably loud enough; flowmeters, dials, gauges, and control identifications easy to see; back lighting on control panels helpful for night viewing.
Cleaning and maintenance	Easy to perform; disassembly and reassembly should follow an uncomplicated, logical order; has easy-to-reach corners and crevices when cleaning.

care: the virtual lack of bed-induced decubiti. Allegorically, good home care means the patient should have the same or even fewer problems that he would have if he were still hospitalized. In theory, the patient should fare better at home. In addition to the fact that the home-care patient is in familiar surroundings, there is an additional sound medical reason for at-home care: no risk of nosocomial infection. Costs of home care are naturally greatly reduced, and that will be briefly discussed in the next section. The overall success of each patient's home-care experience varies with the degree of illness, compliance, family support, and a host of psychosocial factors. In general, the following items are indications that point to a potentially positive home-care experience for all involved:

1. Good predischarge planning by the pulmonary rehabilitation team.

2. Good communication with patient and family by all taking part in the patient's care (primary physician, rehabilitation team, DME dealer, social agencies, and insurance carrier).

3. Ability and willingness by patient and others involved with his health care to be 100% faithful to prescribed routines, medication schedule, equipment cleaning, etc.

4. Compliance, compliance, compliance!

Cost Of Home Care

While it would be difficult to compute a patient's home-care costs to the nearest dollar, fairly accurate and useful comparisons can be made contrasting home care with hospital costs. The now classic South Hills Health Service project in Pittsburgh, Pa., conducted one of the first studies to determine costs of hospitalization vs. home-care costs.[1] A recent update[2] on this project further proved not only the medical necessity, but the cost benefits as well. Respiratory therapy home visitations helped reduce readmission rates and hospital costs. A private study in 1979[3] not only supported the South Hills project, but cited economic incentives to employers to provide a rider (i.e., a clause in a health insurance contract) that would provide at-home and outpatient respiratory care. Another study by the Maryland Medicaid Home Respiratory Support Program echoed the same findings in terms of simplicity of home visitations and large cost reductions.[4]

While such studies almost always show a decrease in hospital stay and concomitant health-care costs, there still seems to be a general reluctance to support this extended form of health care. It is not possible in this book to focus in-depth on these problems. However, the author feels an obligation to apprise the reader of the paradoxes of our health care system that bring about the unnecessary extension of in-hospital care merely to provide like services that can be easily and safely performed on an outpatient and home-care basis. This summation provides only a glimpse of historic and legislative occurrences that have bogged down the collective efforts of health professionals, public agencies, and DME dealers in their efforts to provide cost-effective home health care. The following situations refer specifically to the respiratory care portion of the reimbursement problem. The respiratory therapists' dilemma presents as one of the more unique examples of bureaucratic mindlessness.

1. Lack of recognition by third-party payers that respiratory therapists are professionals and should be accorded the same remunerative privileges as other health professionals.

2. The lack of many health insurance plans, especially those provided to workers in pulmonary-polluting jobs, to provide a clause which covers outpatient and home-care rehabilitative services. This is not necessarily the fault of the insurance carrier; instead, it reflects an unwillingness or lack of foresight by the employer to take on the additional costs of the insurance rider. The employer ends up paying in the end anyway, in the form of medical disability benefits, loss of worker's time, etc.

3. The cutbacks by the federal government on federally funded insurance plans such as Medicare. This has severely limited health care services of a rehabilitative nature.

4. The incalculable amount of fraud and unethical practices by some DME dealers that has projected a sour image upon home care, especially where oxygen usage and related respiratory equipment is used.

5. Indiscriminate ordering of outpatient and home-care services by physicians in an attempt to pacify the patient. Subsequent Medicare, Medicaid

audits uncover this, and as a result, the increased scrutiny may affect patients who really need the service.

6. Legislators who issue promulgations (i.e., orders to federal insurance intermediaries) that cut out or severely restrict allowances for specific services or supplies. (A classic example in 1979 was Transmittal 702, which in its original form would have limited home oxygen usage to only those patients with a 12 hours-a-day *minimum* need for oxygen.)

Even though home care is a logical extension of the patient's in-hospital care, funding may not always be available. In addition to the reasons cited above, lack of an active home-care program may also be due to simply a lack of physician support and insufficient interest by the hospital and community as a whole. Hospitals struggling for health care dollars may be reluctant to support noninpatient or outpatient programs that reduce the number of bed days a patient may be expected to normally accumulate. There is indeed a paradox to this type of thinking: Do hospitals exist to serve the health-care needs of the community, returning citizens to gainful employment, or is their function to increase revenues by overextended hospital stays for the meritorious purpose of buying better health care equipment? Perhaps the patient's employers should be induced to provide an incentive in the form of a donation for every one of its sick employees the hospital speedily returns to gainful employment. This system may be more revenue productive than keeping the patient for an extra day or two.

In addition to the above-mentioned problems, the cost-benefit ratio of freeing up in-hospital staff to perform home care is of paramount concern. Astute hospital administrators and department directors may find the cost of providing home care to its patients is simply not cost-effective. After computing travel time and costs to and from the hospital to the patient's home, along with the health-care worker's salary, the cost-benefit of seeing just one patient becomes foreboding; and there is not necessarily safety in numbers, because a series of trips to other patients' homes in a 1-day period still involves travel time, set-up time, etc. Also, one must figure in the time for social amenities involved with being a "guest" in the patient's home; the traditional coming-and-going greeting system found in the hospital setting does not prevail in the patient's personal surroundings. In the patient's domicile, the health care worker must work more closely and in accordance with the patient's wishes. It can be a stark contrast to the open ward or semiprivate room where the patient is at the mercy of the health professional. (This author will have the reader know that the former is indeed a humbling experience!)

An Alternative to Hospital-Based Home Care

A viable alternative to consider is the concept of having qualified home-care companies provide some or all of the home-care services. This may be especially feasible for hospitals desiring to provide home care or some sort of follow-up on their discharged patients, but lacking the time or funds to do it. This concept may work especially well with the respiratory therapy services required in view of the fact that this profession, as mentioned earlier, finds home-care reimbursement a problem. The reader must not confuse the identity of a home-care consultant with the oxygen and equipment supplier. Many home-care companies now employ respiratory therapists and technicians to do initial oxygen and equipment set-ups in the patient's home. In this capacity, they are relegated to functioning as a highly qualified equipment placement technician only. They do not give any home-care instructions other than that relative to the equipment. The home-care consultant (also a credentialed respiratory therapist), on the other hand, would be giving home-care instructions to the same degree that the hospital-delegated health professional would. He would then write a report to the referring hospital detailing the visit. One very entrepreneurial group in Dayton, Ohio, is investigating the merits of this concept (Respiratory Consultants of Dayton, 3490 Upper Bellbrook Rd., Bellbrook, OH 45305).

Summary

The two members of the in-hospital pulmonary rehabilitation team playing the more active home-care roles are the respiratory therapist and nurse. Their responsibilities may even take on a wider scope, because they must act as the eyes and ears of the other team members not taking an active in-home role.

The patient and his family members also are to take an active role by following the home-care regimen closely and alerting the health professionals of any deviation. Compliance is mandatory on the patient's part if he is to have a succesful at-home experience. The key to assessing the quality of his home care is the infrequency of repeated exacerbations. The patient's psychosocial adjustment is also a monitoring device.

Of paramount importance is the recognition by reimbursement agencies that home care can be cost-effective. In spite of overwhelming proof to this fact, many third-party payers are still reluctant to remunerate these costs. Paradoxically, while home care is cost-effective, it may not prove to be so for the various members rendering the actual in-home care, notably the respiratory therapist. Unfortunately, the therapist's recognition by insurance carriers is minimal or, more often, totally lacking. Concomitant with these problems is the tremendous ignorance by legislators who historically have been indifferent to the role that the respiratory therapy profession plays in the patient's pulmonary care. Testimony to this is the attempted passing of Transmittal 702 in its original form.

As a viable alternative to hospital-provided home care, in view of the cost-effectiveness for the sponsoring hospital, consideration may be given to home-care consultants who can usually provide the care at a more effective, efficient cost-benefit ratio.

Chapter 14 provides an excellent example of home care of a specific type of patient, the *ventilator-dependent* patient, and gives the reader an excellent and in-depth practicum of home care in action. Chapter 14 serves two purposes: (1) to give the reader a beginning-to-end practicum of one category of home care and (2) to concomitantly introduce the reader to a unique facet of home care still in a developing stage, that of in-home care of the ventilator-dependent patient.

References

1. Young W.J.: Third parties and home-care RTs—The frustrating search for a little recognition. *Respir. Therapy,* May/June, 1978.
2. Roselle S.R., D'Amico F.J.: The effect of home respiratory therapy on hospital re-admission rates of patients with chronic pulmonary disease. *Respir. Care* 82:1194, 1982.
3. O'Ryan J.A.: Blue Cross respiratory project. January 1979 (unpublished).
4. Fratto C.A., Flynn J.P.G., Singer R.M.: The Maryland Medicaid Home Respiratory Support Program. A comprehensive approach. *Md. State Med. J.* April 1977, pp. 20–26.

Suggested Reading

1. Colt A.M., Anderson N., Scott H.D., Zimmerman H.: Home health care is good economics. *Nurs. Outlook* 25:632–636, 1977.
2. Malkus B.L.: Respiratory care at home. *Am. J. Nurs.* 76:1789–1791, 1976.
3. May D.F., Kenny W.R.: Pulmonary rehabilitation: Dealing effectively with chronic pulmonary disease. *J. Med. Assoc. Ga.* 69:205, 1980.

14 / Home Ventilator Care

JEFFREY LUCAS, R.R.T.

MECHANICAL VENTILATION in the home has arisen from a variety of influences, the most prominent being as follows:

1. Early diagnosis and treatment of debilitating pulmonary disorders resulting in increased longevity that necessitates extended-care requirements.

2. Committed physicians and health-team members offering appropriate supportive and rehabilitative care to the chronically disabled, making it possible for the patient needing mechanical life support to live at home.

3. Socioeconomic stresses demanding reductions in costs placed on the health care industry.

4. Concerned family members wanting greater access to their separated family members.

5. Recent technologic advancements offering portability, simplicity, versatility, compactness, and improved safety to the home-bound ventilator patient, his caretakers, and his environment. Examples of these advances are the Life Products LP-4 ventilator, battery operated suction equipment, and compact physiologic monitoring systems.

Caring for the patient in need of mechanical support of ventilation in the home is being accomplished on a small scale quite successfully nationwide.[1-8] This patient population will continue to grow as the general medical community and third-party payers come to realize the benefits and observe the rewards offered by this alternative.

The goal in this chapter is to outline the major processes necessary to provide for a successful hospital-to-home transition for the ventilator-dependent patient and his family. This chapter will examine assessments of the patient as a prime candidate for home ventilation, the family as "primary care givers," and a physical view of the home as well as equipment selection and routine care, regular patient follow-up and an in-hospital vs. home-cost comparison for this type of patient.

Identifying the Prime Candidate for
Home Mechanical Ventilation

The majority of patients managed most successfully in the home environment can be identified as "those patients determined clinically unable to support the necessary ventilatory requirement to sustain life." However, this criteria must be met without the presence of acute pulmonary dysfunction, significant oxygenation disorders, and or contributing multiple-organ system failure. In other words, the patient's day-to-day cardiopulmonary status must be of a relatively stable quality without any wide fluctuations that could only be treated by aggressive in-hospital modalities.

Patients meeting with this general clinical premise will offer minimal management problems on a day-to-day basis, which will in turn lessen stress on the patient and the primary care givers.

Three profiles have emerged from the present population of ventilator-dependent patients studied by this author in the home:

1. The patient unable to maintain adequate spontaneous ventilatory function over prolonged time periods.

2. The patient exhibiting stable ventilatory failure associated with prolonged longevity, but requiring continuous mechanical support.

3. The newly diagnosed terminally ill patient demonstrating stable ventilatory failure associated with minimal longevity.

Table 14–1 is a listing of the disorders grouped in each profile.

This is by no means an attempt to pigeonhole prime candidates for mechanical ventilation in the home; it must be stressed that each patient and family be viewed independently. Many other factors will play a role in the final decision-making process, which will be discussed later. At the time a patient is initially being considered as a home-going candidate, the plan should immediately be presented to the family for open discussion. The input of the physician, patient, and family at the onset of the decision-making process can then collectively put into perspective the fears, responsibilities, and expectations of those involved in the anticipated home-care undertaking. All three parties must explore the implications of changing family lifestyles, continuous care, and financial responsibilities, as well as the ultimate course of the disease process. At this time, a collective decision must be made before the next step in the home-going process can be initiated.

Once the physician, patient, and family have decided that the return to home is feasible, an overall assessment of the patient and home is initiated. This would include a summary of the patient's present clinical state, an assessment of the family as primary care givers, and a look at the physical

TABLE 14–1.—PATIENT PROFILE TYPES REQUIRING ASSISTED VENTILATION IN THE HOME

	GROUP DESCRIPTION	DISEASES INVOLVED
Profile 1	Mainly composed of neuromuscular and thoracic wall disorders; particular stage of disease process allows patient certain periods of spontaneous breathing time during day; generally require only nocturnal mechanical support.	Amyotrophic lateral sclerosis Multiple sclerosis Kyphoscoliosis and related chest-wall deformities Diaphragmatic paralysis Myasthenia gravis
Profile 2	Requires continuous mechanical ventilatory support associated with long-term survival rates.	High spinal cord injuries Apneic encephalopathies Severe chronic obstructive lung disease Late-stage muscular dystrophy
Profile 3	Usually returns home at request of patient and family; patient is terminal, life expectancy is short, and patient and family wish to spend remaining time at home; patients usually pose significant management problems in the home due to rapidly deteriorating condition.	Lung cancer End-stage chronic obstructive pulmonary disease

layout of the residence to ensure a safe and efficient environment. Table 14–2 summarizes the primary aspects of the assessment routine.

The primary care giver(s) in the home generally are competent, enthusiastic, trainable family members, but can also be a live-in friend or hired professional personnel. Whatever the case, they must be made aware of the fact that their services will be required on a 24-hour, 7-days-per-week schedule if the patient is in need of continuous mechanical ventilator support. For the patient requiring only nocturnal support, the primary care giver must still be available at all times. This is an awesome undertaking; therefore, plenty of backup professional help and support must be available and accessible prior to instituting home ventilator care.

Home-Care Team Members

Several key health care professionals form the nucleus of the effort to successfully manage the ventilator-dependent patient at home. The professional staff involved in the home-going plans and continued care should include the following:

TABLE 14–2.—SUMMARY OF FUNDAMENTAL ASSESSMENT CRITERIA
NEEDED FOR SUCCESSFUL HOME CARE

1. Competent, trainable family, live-in friend, or dependable professional staff possessing the ability to take over in the absence of family and willing to spend the time required for proper training.
2. Patient willing to go home
3. Family fully understands prognosis and diagnosis.
4. No evidence of acute underlying pulmonary abnormalities.
5. Patient's clinical pulmonary condition stable and free of contributing multiorgan system failure.
6. Family aware of their financial responsibilities.
7. Psychological consult assigned at the time the patient is made to return home.
8. Home environment conducive to returning patient.
9. Electrical facilities are adequate to safely operate all equipment.
10. Patient environment controlled, alleviating drafts during winter months and insuring proper ventilation in warm seasons.
11. Pets and substances that may produce allergic responses for the patient removed or controlled.
12. Adequate equipment cleaning and storage space provided.

THE PRIMARY PHYSICIAN.—He will receive regular input from the primary care givers and the professionals involved in the continuing care. The physician decides on care-plan changes via this input (e.g., changes in medication usage, ventilator setting changes, etc.). He should also be actively involved in the home-going instructions and planning in order to be familiar with all aspects of the patient's circumstances. If the primary physician is not a pulmonary specialist, then one should be involved on a consultation basis.

THE PSYCHOLOGICAL CONSULTANT.—It is imperative that not only the patient, but the family as well, be availed of the services of a pyschological consultant. Some patients and their families cope exceedingly well with the changes imposed on their lifestyles. However, others do not, and professional psychological help can relieve intrafamily conflicts, guilt, and other problems arising with their new responsibilities as the caretakers of a handicapped family member. It is easy to sympathize with the lay person who, within the time frame of approximately one month, has traversed from the role of visitor in a completely unfamiliar environment to one offering the complete care and responsibility to a family member on mechanical life support. This emotional stress will dramatically affect the lives of those involved with the day-to-day care of the home ventilator patient.

THE RESPIRATORY THERAPIST.—The therapist should be involved as instructor, follow-up person, and consultant on a continuing basis. Preferably, the same therapist should instruct the primary care givers on ventilator and circuit function, tracheostomy tube care, suctioning, etc. Many times, one therapist with experience in this area will be asked to coordinate and implement the entire home-going process, from initial assessment and instruction to transporting the patient home and providing the follow-up. Maintaining the same personnel involvement from start to finish is important. This continuity allows the patient and family to gain confidence and improves communications with all involved.

THE NURSE.—Primary nursing care should be implemented at the time the patient is selected as a candidate for home ventilator care. This will ensure continuity of care and also offer another consultant to the family over the course of in-hospital training and preparation. Those nurses assigned to the patient on a regular daily basis should either attend all family instructional sessions or actively participate in the instruction so conflicting information is not disseminated to the family. The key to a rapid and successful training program for the lay family is (1) keep it *simple*, (2) *rehearse*, and (3) *reinforce*. This can only be accomplished when all personnel involved are on the same track. The nurse is helpful in providing suggestions to ease daily care routines, skin care, vital sign records, medication usage and effectiveness, and acting as a liason to the primary physician.

THE SOCIAL SERVICE OR HOME-CARE PLANNER.—This individual is a very important member to the home-care plan. Arrangements with a reputable home-care and equipment supplier must be made; the financial burden of equipment and professional personnel (if needed) can be dramatically lessened by the discharge planner who investigates all avenues of financial aid to the family. The discharge planner can also arrange for needed community services to be made available to the patient and family. These services may include providing transportation, visiting nursing personnel, occasional meals, socializing, or whatever the particular situation may require to lessen the burden on the primary care givers.

THE HOME-CARE AND EQUIPMENT SUPPLIER.—The supplier must be a reputable firm that employs trained respiratory therapists who can advise which type of oxygen system (if needed) will be most efficient, economical, and safe for the particular mechanical ventilator being used. The supplier must also be a full-service company, able to supply and service all of the patient's equipment needs (e.g., mechanical ventilator, tracheostomy dressings, oxygen supply, etc.). This will relieve the family of any further confusion from having to call more than one supplier when a piece of equipment needs service or supplies need replenishing. The home-care supplier must have respiratory therapists on staff who are available for 24-hour call, 7 days a week, for response to any mechanical or oxygen system failure that may have to be repaired or replaced. Costs vary widely among home suppliers, and this should enter as a consideration, also; however, it should not preclude the prerequisite of good service performed by qualified personnel.

Indeed, it is important that all personnel involved in the initial instruction, discharge planning, and continuing follow-up be knowledgeable, qualified individuals in the aspects of home care and mechanical ventilation relative to their responsibilities.

Primary Care Givers: The Family

There should ideally be more than one person in the family designated as the primary care giver; this will allow for family members to break from the routine and stress of caring for that individual. The patient on mechanical support of ventilation in the hospital, specifically in critical care units, experiences sleep and sensory deprivation along with poor nutritional supplementation.[5] In the home, the same phenomena can happen to the primary care givers if there is not sufficient help to allow for personal time off. This is an important facet to be monitored during regular follow-up visits.

Not all ventilator-dependent patients at home require 24-hour support or care. A large percentage require only nocturnal support and lead very active, relatively normal daytime lives, and for the most part care for themselves and their own equipment. Even in the case of nocturnal-only ventilator support, family members should still be required to attend instructional sessions. This is necessary to provide for effective assistance in case of emergencies or if the patient requires help during an exacerbation. This is the ideal home-ventilator patient-family relationship. This group of patients then experience little or no management problems, family stress and anxiety is at a minimum, and the patient can continue on with daily living almost totally unencumbered. These patients are examples of those listed in profile 1.

Patient types defined previously in profiles 2 and 3 will require much more time and effort and will encounter many more problems.

The patient profiled in the third category can be an exhaustive task for the care givers. In certain instances, such as the older man with terminal, end-stage lung cancer, the family may wish to bring him home for what time is remaining, no matter what the cost in terms of time and money. The initial assessment may reveal this patient is not the ideal candidate for home ventilator care, but how does one deny their wishes? Do we as suppliers of health care and services even have the legal right to say no? This patient group will at times tax the resources of every member of the health team involved. It must be emphasized here that a successful home situation rests on complete and thorough in-hospital preparation.

The family must also be made totally aware of the patient's diagnosis and prognosis. If the family is not fully aware of the patient's limitations and probable continued regression of physical state, depending upon the disease entity, false hopes, despair, and depression are sometimes observed. This may be followed by resentment for the entire situation and all participating members of the team. In situations such as this, the family may also spend a great deal of money on unnecessary accessory equipment such as exercycles, treadmills, and the like. The fire of resentment is fueled when excess monies are spent fruitlessly in an already-expensive undertaking.

Clinical Profile of Ideal Home Ventilator Patient

A very important aspect of the initial assessment is to determine the patient's clinical stability. It is difficult to define clinical stability in a patient requiring life support with a progressive disease entity. However, most successful patient management situations in the home have exhibited the following predischarge characteristics:

1. Two to 4 weeks of relatively unchanging ventilatory parameters resulting in minimal fluctuations of acid-base and blood gas status.

2. Two to 4 weeks of minimal demonstrable shunt requiring a fractional inspired oxygen concentration (FI_{O2}) of 35% or less to correct.

3. Two to 4 weeks of nondeteriorating spontaneous ventilatory parameters (tidal volume, spontaneous ventilatory frequency, minute volume, vital capacity, negative inspiratory force).

4. Minimal use of diuretics, chronotropic, or ionotropic agents, afterload reduction agents, or vasopressors (extreme in-home management problems can arise with contributing multiorgan system failure).

5. No evidence of acute underlying pulmonary abnormalities, i.e., infection, pleural effusions, atelectasis, etc.

6. Last, but not least, proper tracheostomy tube cuff maintenance should be closely observed. Tracheal dilation and tracheal-esophageal fistulas resulting from improper cuff care present the same inordinate management problems in the home as they do in the hospital. Food and medication aspiration and aerophagia resulting in abdominal distension are recurrent hazards that can sorely disrupt an otherwise successful in-home course.

Cost Considerations

As early as possible during the in-hospital assessment routine, the family must be exposed to the cost considerations related to this endeavor. This point should actually be discussed during the early decision-making process with the physician, patient, and family. Financial obligations will definitely play a major role in determining the feasibility of the project. Table 14–3 is an in-home vs. hospital-cost comparison. Regardless what the insurance

TABLE 14–3 HOME VS. IN-HOSPITAL COST COMPARISON FOR VENTILATOR CARE*

| | AVERAGE MONTHLY COST | | |
	HOME CARE† ($)	IN-HOSPITAL‡ ($)	IN-HOSPITAL‡ ($)
Patient A	875	21,461	715
Patient B	1,013	23,353	778
Patient C	1,175	27,950	932
Patient D	1,004	21,397	713
Patient E	892	17,370	579

*All costs calculated from actual patient billing statements of expenses incurred between March 1979 and October 1982. Only 5 of 25 patients reported here because of extreme similarities in charges. Data courtesy of T & M Oxygen Co., Inc., Cleveland.

†Figures represent total cost of replenishable medical supplies such as gloves, suction catheters, and oxygen plus rented equipment (e.g., ventilator, wheelchair, bedside commode, etc.). Expenditures not consistent from family to family, such as hired nursing care or physician visits, are not reported.

‡Hospital room charge (ward and nursing services) plus respiratory therapy costs (ventilator, oxygen, arterial blood sampling, bronchopulmonary hygiene, and aerosol therapy if itemized). Figures do not include physician or procedure charges for services such as radiography, laboratory, etc.

reimbursement situation may be for the patient, it is a rare instance in which the third-party payer will pay 100% of the expenses incurred. The family is almost always responsible for a portion of that cost, which can be staggering, depending upon insurance coverage.

A close approximation of the actual financial outlay from the patient and family should be determined before any further steps are taken in the process of bringing the patient home. It is unfair to allow the patient and family to believe that third-party payers will reimburse most of the cost. The burden of assuming that portion of the expenses not covered by third-party payers is a relative situation from family to family, but can be usually assumed to be of a serious monetary import to most families. Actual figures, reimbursement, and cost-commitments from third-party payers and suppliers should be obtained and presented to the family at the very beginning, prior to any actual home-care arrangements being made.

Evaluation Of The Home

Once the patient assessment has been completed, an evaluation of the home is performed. Emphasis is placed on the electrical facilities to determine adequacy for safe operation of all equipment that will be placed in the home. Table 14–4 lists common electrically operated medical equipment and their amperage requirements. A number of the items listed in Table 14–4 may be operating simultaneously, which means that the electrical circuitry must be adequate to supply the amperage draw at peak-use periods. Another requirement is that all grounded electrical outlets to be

used for any of the medical devices be placed on specially designated 15-
to 20-amp circuits with their own fuse box. This will avoid any power over-
load or outages on that circuit from overused or faulty household appli-
ances.

Observation of the patient's room and other general-care areas where the
patient may be is important to determine ideal placement of electrical outlets, space requirements for equipment and supply storage, and ease of
movement for patient and family. Often, dining rooms or living rooms are
converted to patient-care areas in the home. Equipment needs will play a
large role in determining space requirements. The complete patient management system should be envisioned at this time. Will one "H" cylinder
of oxygen be sufficient to supply the patients needs over an appropriate
time period, or will the patient require a large 40-gal liquid reservoir with
five manifolded "H" cylinders as emergency backup? Where will the oxygen be stored? From which entrance will it be delivered? Where will the
gas connections for the primary and backup ventilators be installed? Will
the patient need an electrically operated hospital bed, a bedside commode,
or a walker? These are only a few example questions that must be answered. Pets or substances that may produce allergic responses for the
patient must be removed or effectively controlled. The room or care area
that has been selected must be draft-free during the winter months, while
provisions for proper ventilation and air conditioning in warm seasons must
be ensured. Adequate areas for equipment processing must be identified.

TABLE 14–4.—AMPERAGE REQUIREMENTS FOR COMMONLY PLACED HOME-
CARE EQUIPMENT

Bennet MA-1 Ventilator	4.5 amps
(Puritan-Bennett Corporation)	
LP-4 Ventilator – 110 Volt Operation	3.0 amps
(Life Products, Inc.)	
EconO$_2$ Oxygen Concentrator	7.0 amps
(Mountain Medical Equipment, Inc.)	
DeVO$_2$ Model 965 Oxygen Concentrator	10.0 amps
(DevilBiss Corporation)	
Bennett Model AP-5 IPPB Unit	1.6 amps
(Puritan-Bennett Corporation)	
Cascade 1 Humidifier Heater	1.2 amps
(Puritan-Bennett Corporation)	
DevilBiss Model 35B Ultrasonic Nebulizer	0.75 amps
(DevilBiss Corporation)	
Timeter Model 2000 Air Compressor	12.0 amps
(Timeter Instrument Corporation)	
Electric Hospital Bed	3.5 amps
(Hill-Rom Company)	
Suction Machine	1.6 amps
(Gomco Surgical Manufacturing Corp.)	

These areas should have some degree of counter space for disassembling and reassembling the equipment that requires disinfection, sterilization, and reuse. Drying and storage areas for processed tubing and miscellaneous parts will also be needed. The home should be inspected for proper screening to limit invasion of houseflies, mosquitoes, and other insects that may result in clean equipment contamination and infect or annoy the patient.

Once the patient has been identified as a home-bound candidate, the care givers chosen, and the home inspected, training sessions can be introduced.

Instructional Routine

Thorough training for the family is essential to producing a successful care and management experience in the home. This is the opportunity for the family to build self-confidence. They must be assured they can accomplish the task and correct commonly encountered problems on their own. Expect most patients and their families to approach the early instruction with fear and anxiety. This can be alleviated by keeping the directions simple and concise. The first meeting should consist of an organized breakdown of the entire training program. Reference and summary material should be given to the care givers at the onset of instruction. This will offer insight as to what will be expected of them throughout and an opportunity to discuss and review the material in private. Table 14–5 is an example of

TABLE 14–5.—PATIENT AND FAMILY EDUCATION CHECKLIST*

I. Ventilator
_____ Description of ventilator function and basic function of each control.
_____ Detailed explanation of high and low pressure alarms; what each alarm indicates and what to troubleshoot.
_____ Family must memorize the following causes:
Activation of high pressure alarm
1. Kink in tubing
2. Secretion accumulation indicating a need for suctioning
3. Water accumulation in tubing
4. Patient coughing
5. Gradual increases in peak airway pressure over a period of days may indicate pulmonary infection (see pulmonary infection).
Activation of low pressure alarm
1. Patient disconnect
2. Malfunctioning exhalation valve
3. Loose fitting on humidifier or nebulizer
4. Leak in circuitry at tubing connections
5. Holes or splits in tubing
6. Malfunctioning tracheostomy tube cuff
_____ Detailed description of tubing circuitry: how to disassemble and reassemble complete ciruit, including humidifier.
_____ Must be able to test for circuit integrity before each use.
_____ Must be able to reassemble and troubleshoot circuit with deliberate mal-

functions placed by therapist (e.g., missing parts, added parts, missing exhalation valve diaphragm, etc.).

_____ Family must wash and/or glove hands before manipulating circuit.

_____ Describe frequency and routine for cleaning procedure as follows:

1. Circuit to be cleaned every third day.
2. Completely disassemble circuit and humidifier; wash in detergent followed by thorough rinse.
3. Soak all components in a 1:3 white vinegar and water solution for 20 minutes, or use chemical germicide as instructed.
4. Rinse and dry completely; bag or cover until used.

_____ Identify location of filter(s) that must be cleaned or replaced.

II. Suctioning

_____ Instruct on proper sterile or clean technique.

_____ Patient must be manually ventilated with manual resuscitator between each pass of the suction catheter.

_____ Description and use of suction machine.

_____ Disassembly of resuscitation bag for cleaning, which will be the same frequency as the ventilator circuit.

_____ Proper disposal of glove and catheter in bag-lined receptacle to be emptied daily.

III. Tracheal Stoma Care

_____ Frequency must be minimum of once daily.

_____ Glove hands after washing.

_____ Remove old dressing and using a 50% hydrogen peroxide and normal saline solution, swab entire area of stoma to remove excessive drainage and/or secretions that may be present.

_____ Check stomal area for signs of infection or irritation.

_____ Optional: If stoma site is reddened, irritated, or consistently moist due to presence of pulmonary secretions, a Betadine ointment may be applied before placing the new dressing.

_____ Change tracheal ties if soiled.

IV. Signs of Pulmonary Infection

_____ Gradual sustained increases in peak airway pressure.

_____ Increase in body temperature.

_____ Increase in number of times patient must be suctioned per day.

_____ Change in color and/or consistency of secretions.

_____ Foul odor of secretions.

V. Tracheostomy Tube Care

_____ Clean technique with gloved hands.

_____ Instruct to cleanse inner cannula utilizing a 50% solution of hydrogen peroxide and normal saline as soak; scrub with cannula brush followed by clean rinse in normal saline.

VI. Cuff Inflation and Deflation Technique

_____ (Fenestrated tube) Instruct on cuff deflation and tube plugging technique.

_____ (Bivona tube) instruct on daily deflation routine to check cuff integrity.

_____ For inflatable cuffs in general, stress accuracy in replacing required sealing volume in cuff after deflating.

VII. Vital Signs

_____ Instruct on pulse taking and stress importance of pulse if patient is receiving periodic aerosolized bronchodilators; record patient's baseline pulse for future reference.

_____ Instruct family on counting spontaneous respiratory rate; record patient's baseline for future reference.

_____ Instruct in performing blood pressure measurements; record patient's baseline for future reference.

*Courtesy of T & M Oxygen Co., Inc. Cleveland.

a checklist that summarizes the required instructional goals for the family.

A participatory, hands-on approach to the equipment from the beginning can be an effective route to tempering apprehension. Allow 1 to 2 days between each scheduled training period. This will give the family time to assimilate and practice new techniques presented to them. Each successive meeting should begin with a practical review of the techniques and information given during the previous session. The hospital nursing staff should be kept abreast of the family's progress so they may allow them to perform those care duties in the hospital. Allowing the care givers to participate in the care routine provides for continuing reinforcement, practice of skills, and offers an opportunity for the family to gain confidence and experience in managing the various problems that may arise. Whenever possible, the family should be given the actual equipment to take home with them so they may practice assembling and operating such items as tubing circuitry, suction machines, tracheostomy tubes, and tracheostomy tube care kits.

The care givers should be trained to change the patient's tracheostomy tube whenever necessary. By doing so, expensive trips to the hospital, outpatient facility charges, and the unwieldy task of transporting the patient for what is actually a relatively quick and simple procedure can be eliminated. The family should also possess the ability to place a new tube in the event of an airway emergency.

Avoid setting a mandatory discharge date to work toward; the in-hospital instruction should not be hurried in order to ensure adequate preparation. Optimally, when the instructional routine is completed, a 24- to 48-hour period is arranged so the family may live in with the patient at the hospital. During this time, the family should be permitted to offer complete around-the-clock care for the patient. This experience gives the patient and family a good overall perspective of their recently acquired abilities as well as the opportunity to resolve any final questions or concerns.

Final procedural assessments are performed by the prescribing physician, respiratory therapist, and nurse to determine the care givers' skills in equipment troubleshooting and patient care regimen. These assessments will offer a comprehensive view of the family's abilities to the professional home-going team. Chapter 11 discusses patient education in depth.

Ancillary Equipment Selection

The task of selecting the appropriate equipment for the patient is not difficult if one is simply listing supply needs for the home that parallel his in-hospital supplies. Generally speaking, what the patient is utilizing daily in the hospital is what he will need at home. However, situations and supplies not seen daily in the hospital will often pose logistical problems in the home. For instance, if the patient is ambulatory and does not require continuous mechanical support, there may be a need for a portable ventilator with a self-contained or portable power source. Will the patient be spending extended periods of time away from home? If so, he may require a portable suction unit with battery-operated capabilities. Oxygen systems, when required, pose a number of logistic questions. What type of oxygen system must be installed to meet the patient's needs? How and where will the oxygen system be placed? And how will the oxygen and humidity be provided from room to room when the patient is off the ventilator? The qualified and experienced home-care and equipment supplier is best suited to offer solutions to these questions. These situations must be presented to the supplier early to allow for sufficient preparation time. Figure 14–1 depicts a relatively complex oxygen supply system that was placed in a patient's home. This patient required an inspired oxygen concentration of 70% with a corresponding average minute volume of 18 L. In addition, he lived in a remote area approximately a 1½-hour drive from the supplier. Late in the patient's course, he was requiring almost 200,000 L of oxygen per week!

The family should be given a complete listing of all the equipment and supplies that will be placed in the home so provisions for proper storage can be made before the patient goes home. Table 14–6 is an actual equipment and supply listing. Although this listing appears lengthy, it is by no means extraordinary for the home-bound ventilator-dependent patient.

Ventilator Selection

In this author's experience with 25 home ventilator patients, the most commonly used ventilators have been the time-cycled, volume-controlled Life Products LP-4 and the volume-cycled Bennett MA-1. Other ventilators that have been used include the Emerson 3-PV Post-Op, the Bennett PR-2, and the Bird Mark 7. All of the above ventilators are classified as positive pressure units that require attachment to the patient via an artificial airway. Others reporting in the literature are enjoying similar success using negative pressure ventilators such as the Cuirass-type units, which do not require attachment to artificial airways.[2, 4] The use of these devices, however, is restricted to patients with little intrinsic pulmonary involvement and relatively normal chest configurations.

There are a large number of important variables that must be considered when choosing a ventilator for home use. Some of the major considerations include the following:

1. SAFETY.—The ventilator must be mechanically dependable over long periods of time. It should be UL approved and safe to operate in an oxy-

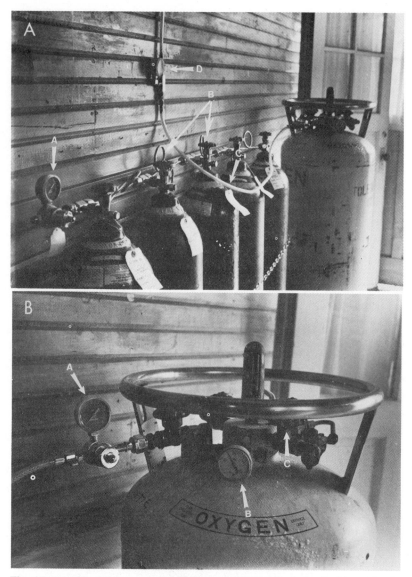

Fig 14–1.—A, oxygen supply system placed against an inside wall of attached garage at the patient's home. The liquid oxygen vessel was the primary oxygen source for the patient on an MA-1 ventilator. The manifolded compressed gas cylinders were placed as an emergency backup gas supply for the ventilator. Shown here is the 50-psi pressure-reducing valve for the oxygen cylinder bank *(A)*, copper manifold tubing for connecting compressed gas cylinders in series *(B)*, oxygen supply line *(C)*, and oxygen supply line pressure-monitoring gauge *(D)*. **B,** 50-psi reducing valve for liquid oxygen reservoir *(A)*, internal vessel contents pressure gauge *(B)*, and manually operated vessel vent valve *(C)*.

TABLE 14–6.—TYPICAL DISCHARGE EQUIPMENT AND SUPPLY LISTING

A. Primary ventilator
   1. LP-4 ventilator
   2. Manual resuscitator
   3. Three complete patient tubing circuits
   4. Replacement ventilator filters
   5. Daily flow sheets
   6. Extra humidifier (cascade or condensor type)
B. Backup ventilator
   1. Bennett PR-2 ventilator (or similar pneumatically operated unit)
   2. PR-2 patient tubing circuit
   3. Manifolded compressed air cylinders
C. Suction equipment
   1. Suction machine
   2. Extension suction tubing
   3. Suction catheters
   4. Clean gloves
   5. Spare collection bottle
D. Tracheostomy supplies
   1. Spare tracheostomy tubes
   2. Tracheostomy tube dressings
   3. Sterile tracheostomy tube care kits
   4. Sterile water soluble lubricant
   5. Syringes
   6. Sterile gloves
   7. Betadine ointment
   8. Tracheostomy tube ties
   9. Sterile cotton swabs
E. Oxygen source. Depending upon each patient situation, the oxygen source may be compressed gas cylinders, the oxygen concentrator, or liquid oxygen reservoirs. Dictates of the patient-care requirements at home may also necessitate a combination of these systems.
F. Supplemental airway humidity
   1. Portable table or pedestal-mounted cascade humidifier and heater.
   2. Twenty- or 50-ft lengths of 5/16-in. inside diameter, small-bore connecting tubing for air and oxygen bleed-in to humidifier (50-ft, small-bore tubing will necessitate the use of pressure-compensated flowmeters)
   3. Air compressor
   4. Oxygen source (if needed)
   5. Tracheostomy humidity or aerosol collars
   6. Large-bore aerosol tubing
   7. Condensation drainage bags
G. Miscellaneous
   1. Hospital bed
   2. Overbed table
   3. Patient communication aid (e.g., bell, buzzer, intercom, etc.).
   4. Stethoscope
   5. Sphygmomanometer
   6. Commode or urinal
   7. Emergency phone number listing
   8. Plastic bag-lined, covered waste receptacle
   9. Cold chemical disinfectant or white vinegar

gen-enriched environment. The controls should be tamper-proof by children that may live in or visit the patient's home, and it must incorporate alarm systems appropriate to the situation.

2. RELIABILITY.—The preset parameters should not fluctuate over a prolonged operating period or change due to extraneous influences such as circuit type, patient positioning, or varying lung or chest-wall conditions.

3. POWER SOURCE.—If the ventilator is pneumatically driven, it must be remembered that gas sources in the home are not as limitless as when used in the hospital. If the unit is electrically operated, the rate of power consumption should be known. Depending upon the circumstance, arrangements may have to be made for either a backup ventilator or standby power source in the event of a mechanical or electrical failure.

4. EASE OF OPERATION.—An excess of unnecessary alarms and controls can confuse the patient and family. The controls should be well marked and calibrated; if not, a simple problem may become difficult to correct by telephone as well as add complexity to the initial training sessions. All filters that are to be changed on a regular basis must be easily accessible, and the patient circuit should be simple, lightweight, and easy to troubleshoot.

5. VERSATILITY.—As mentioned previously, in situations where the patient does not require continuous ventilatory support, the ventilator should be able to travel with the patient. This could mean anything from a wheelchair to a commercial airliner. The unit must also offer appropriate ventilatory modes to meet with changing patient support and comfort requirements.

6. COST.—Exotic critical care capabilities (that may be unnecessary for in-home ventilator use) or excessive gas use will certainly increase the cost. However, an inexpensive ventilator may actually become less cost-effective if it requires additional operating or monitoring equipment. If the ventilator is carefully chosen to fit the specific needs of each patient, then the cost factor will usually be found justifiable for that situation.

The decision to place a backup ventilator in the home will be based upon the individual patient's requirements because not all patients will require an emergency unit. Patients are generally set up with a secondary unit if it is believed the patient would be in danger due to electrical failure or malfunction of the primary unit. To assess for this need, a number of factors are considered, including (1) the number of hours per day on ventilatory support, (2) the inspired oxygen concentration, (3) the availability and response time of the local emergency squad or ambulance service, and (4) the distance from the nearest hospital and equipment supplier.

Figure 14–2 is an example of a backup ventilator with a reserve power source for the unit. The primary unit is a Life Products LP-4, which incorporates its own internal battery for short operating periods (1 to 1½ hours) during power outages. This does not exempt the unit from mechanical failures, thus the need for the secondary ventilator.

Proper equipment selection and advanced planning for emergencies will decrease or eliminate unnecessary trips to the home for minor problems or last-minute deliveries. This can also be an immeasurable aid in adding to the family's confidence, knowing they are equipped and possess the ability to manage most unexpected situations.

Equipment Decontamination and Infection Control

Decontamination of respiratory therapy equipment and careful adherence to infection-control procedures are vital aspects of mechanical venti-

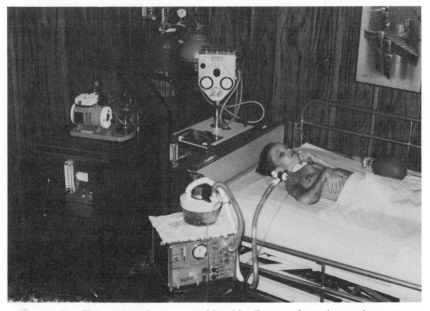

Fig 14–2.—This patient lives a considerable distance from the equipment supplier and requires mechanical support for the major portion of the day, thus the decision to place the secondary Bennett PR-2 ventilator. The patient spends several hours per day off the ventilator. During these periods of spontaneous ventilation, the patient must receive heated, humidified gas with an oxygen concentration of 30%, thus the need for the air compressor and oxygen concentrator. The air compressor is also used to power the secondary ventilator in the event of mechanical failure of the primary unit. The compressed air and oxygen cylinders are placed in case of electrical power failure.

lation in the home. While there are no hard data, it is logical to assume that a patient at home is at less risk from infection than while hospitalized. Nosocomial pneumonia is the third-most-common nosocomial infection and is the most frequent death-related infection occurring in the hospital.[9] Because a large percentage of these infections can be linked to cross-contamination, a well-managed patient at home will be able to avoid such infections. By following proper procedures and decontamination techniques, the incidence of rehospitalization due to pulmonary infection can be minimized. Table 14–7 illustrates the fact that proper training and strict adherence to the decontamination routine will prove effective in preventing pulmonary infections at home.

The areas of infection control that are of prime concern for any ventilator-dependent patient can be roughly categorized into two areas: (1) aseptic procedural techniques, which include tracheostomy tube and stoma care

TABLE 14–7.—COMPARISON OF TOTAL
DAYS SPENT ON MECHANICAL VENTILATOR
AT HOME VS. NUMBER OF HOSPITAL
READMISSION DAYS EXPERIENCED FOR
TREATMENT OF ACQUIRED PULMONARY
INFECTION*

PATIENT	TOTAL HOME-CARE DAYS	TOTAL HOSPITAL READMISSION DAYS
A	405	8
B	133	0
C	1,284	0
D	20	0
E	227	13
F	716	15
G	725	0
H	210	0
I	329	0
J	507	0
K	134	11
L	164	0
M	137	0
N	313	0
O	283	0
P	1,144	0
Q	245	0
R	457	0
S	466	17
T	188	0
U	782	0
V	43	0
Total	8,912	64

*Figures shown represent an average 0.7% hospital readmission rate for treatment of pulmonary infection acquired at home. Data courtesy of T & M Oxygen Co., Inc., Cleveland.

and suctioning and (2) equipment decontamination of such items as humidification systems, patient circuits, and the ventilator itself. The majority of airway procedures such as tracheostomy-tube cleaning, stomal cleaning, and suctioning are instructed as being "clean" techniques as opposed to "sterile" techniques, per se. Thorough hand washing and the use of clean gloves before any airway manipulation occurs is taught to the family. The use of sterile gloves is unnecessary and expensive. Sterile disposable suction catheters are required for use during each suctioning attempt. Sterile and draped conditions are mandated only during tracheostomy tube-change procedures in the home. Inner cannula cleansing of the tracheostomy tube is also performed as a clean technique, and the solution used is one of 1:1 hydrogen peroxide and distilled water yielding a 50% solution. Distilled water is also required as a suction catheter rinse and for use in all humidification devices.

Decontamination of all reusable respiratory therapy equipment such as ventilator circuitry, aerosol tubing, nebulizers, and humidifiers is performed every 3 days with an initial washing in a nonresidue-forming household detergent, then is rinsed thoroughly and followed by soaking in a 2% white vinegar and distilled water solution (a 1:3-part dilution). There has been some controversy in the literature regarding the effectiveness of vinegar for use as a disinfecting agent in the home.[7, 10] Although it has worked well for the patients sent home in this author's experience, the use of a double-quaternary ammonium compound that has become increasingly popular and available for the home patient has been recently recommended. The double-and triple-quaternary ammonium compounds have proved to be cheaper to use than vinegar and more effective against gram-negative and gram-positive organisms than a vinegar and water solution.[7]

The exterior surfaces of the ventilator can be kept clean with any commercially available broad-spectrum germicide or a 70% ethyl alcohol solution. All filters on the unit are to be changed at the frequency recommended by the manufacturer. The family is taught to recognize the early signs and symptoms of a respiratory tract infection, and if such a situation arises, the physician is contacted immediately. A sputum sample is obtained for culture and sensitivity, and the appropriate antibiotic is prescribed (if necessary) and administered at home.

Regularly cleaned and properly stored equipment in the home is not at all a difficult task, but if not performed properly or at the prescribed intervals, the result may be recurrent hospitalizations.

Community Services

A multitude of community services are available to the patient and his family. The services appropriate to the patient's and family's needs should be utilized.

Before the patient is discharged, the family should communicate with their local electric company, emergency squad or ambulance service, and the fire department. The electric company will appropriate priority service to the patient at home requiring life support equipment in the event of a power failure. Those services can range from supplying a portable generator for restoring temporary power to awarding rate discounts. The nearest ambulance service or community rescue squad should be notified prior to the patient returning home. At this time, arrangements should be made for them to visit the home the day the patient returns to visualize the physical layout of the home, the patient's condition (e.g., bed-confined, tracheostomy tube, need for suction equipment, etc.), various equipment being used, and the oxygen system and its location in the home. By actually visiting the home and observing the patient's environment, the emergency service personnel and fire department can best tailor their response and services to any potential crisis.

In many instances, due to the nature of the disease process and medical management requirements, the home-bound ventilator-dependent patient may be leaving a large tertiary care institution or major referral center that is not always close to home. When the patient returns home, the family physician and respiratory therapy personnel at the local hospital should be informed of the patient's circumstance in case he needs immediate emergency attention.

Follow-Up And Continuing Care

The actual follow-up and continued observance of the patient and care givers actually begins before the patient is sent home. The equipment and supplies should be brought to the home a day or two before the patient is discharged. This practice will allow the family to organize the care area and devise a scheduled care routine. Once the equipment and supplies are in place, the family usually has additional questions regarding care practices and equipment operation.

The day the patient returns home, it is essential that personnel from the home-care team be present; this is usually the respiratory therapist and/or the nurse. The team member(s) present should stay until the patient and family feel comfortable, knowing that all systems are operable and the patient is safe. Apprehension on the part of the patient and family is usually visible at this time. Although the care givers felt secure in their responsibilities within the confines of the hospital, it is a different atmosphere at home without dozens of trained personnel available on request. The first week will usually require daily phone checks and possibly two or three visits until the family begins to become more independent.

In this author's experience, it has been found that sending a therapist to

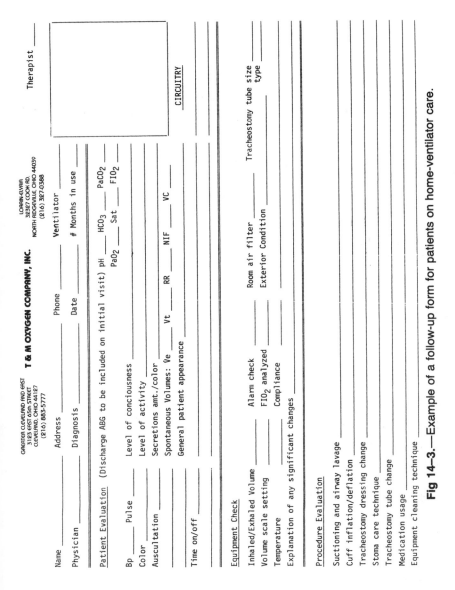

Fig 14–3.—Example of a follow-up form for patients on home-ventilator care.

the patient's home for routine supply deliveries whenever possible can be advantageous in two respects: (1) The home is visited unannounced, providing a more realistic view of intrafamily relations and general care conditions, and (2) visits by qualified personnel are more frequent, thereby improving accessibility to the home-care team for the care givers.

Formal monthly visits to the home are made to furnish records pertaining to the progression (or regression) of the patient's ventilatory status and overall physical condition, vital signs, and total-care routine. Figure 14–3 is an example of a follow-up form.

A ventilator flow sheet is also supplied for the patient. This flow sheet identifies each control on the ventilator. The patient or care giver is instructed to observe each control setting and record this on the form at least once daily. This directs someone in the household to ensure all ventilator controls are set properly each day. The flow sheet is also a reference for substitute home-team members or on-call personnel that are not completely familiar with the prescribed settings. Recording of equipment cleaning dates, changes in secretion color and consistency, and airway-pressure changes are also recorded on the flow sheet.

In the event the patient lives in an outlying area or a significant distance from where he was discharged, it is advisable to acquire the services of a local therapist who will be available to the patient and family for immediate emergencies.

The psychological concerns that are often observed to be associated with ventilator-dependent patients and their families may be far more frequent and serious than any other problems. Denial and depression often displayed by the patient, along with feelings of despair, guilt, and resentment generated by the family, may combine to create serious conflicts within the home. These should be noted by the home-care therapist, nurse, or other outside care givers and reported to the physician.

Summary

Providing the opportunity for ventilator-dependent patients and their families to return home to live in warm and familiar surroundings can be an exhilarating and rewarding experience. The technical ability exists to send this group of patients home safely and comfortably.

Hopefully, more physicians, technical professional personnel, and third-party payers will realize the humanity associated with sending home the patient who requires ventilatory life support. Young people camping and visiting amusement parks and the elderly spending time with their spouses and grandchildren must certainly outweigh inflexible reimbursement schedules and sterile institutional life. The ultimate goal when sending patients home under these circumstances is to *enhance* life, not simply support or prolong it. However, as greater numbers of patients and their families are availed this new option, it is extremely important that they realize the comprehensive responsibilities associated with this type of home care.

References

1. Banaszak E.F., Travers H., Frazier M., et al.: Home ventilator care. *Respir. Care* 26:1262, 1981.
2. Alexander M.A., Johnson E.W., Petty J., et al.: Mechanical ventilation of patients with late stage Duchenne muscular dystrophy: Management in the home. *Arch. Phys. Med. Rehabil.* 60:289, 1979.
3. Lehner W.E., Ballard I.M., Figueroa W.G., et al: Home care utilizing a ventilator in a patient with amyotrophic lateral sclerosis. *J. Fam. Pract.* 10:39, 1980.
4. Holtackers T.R., Loosbrock L.M., Gracey D.R.: The use of the chest cuirass in respiratory failure of neurologic origin. *Respir. Care* 27:271, 1982.
5. Schraeder, B.D.: A creative approach to caring for the ventilator-dependent child. *Matern. Child Nurs. J.* 4:165, 1979.
6. Sivak E.D., Gipson W.T., Hanson E.R.: Long-term management of respiratory failure in amyotrophic lateral sclerosis. *Ann. Neurol.* 12:18, 1982.
7. Fleig C.P.: Double quats disinfectant alternative to vinegar. *Rx. Home Care* 4:37–46, 1982.
8. Feldman J., Tuteur P.G.: Mechanical ventilation: from hospital intensive care to home. *Heart Lung* 11:162, 1982.
9. Simmons B.P., Wong E.S.: Guidelines for prevention of nosocomial pneumonia and guideline ranking scheme: Hospital infections program. Atlanta, Center for Infectious Diseases, Centers for Disease Control, 1982.
10. Assembly for Comprehensive Respiratory Care (ACRC), American Lung Association of Orange County, Calif.: Statement regarding cleaning of home-based respiratory therapy equipment.

15 / Audiovisuals and Print Media; Aids and Organizations

JERRY A. O'RYAN, B.S., R.R.T.

THIS SECTION includes sources of information that augment the rehabilitation practitioner's efforts to teach patients about their lung disease in order for them to actively participate in their care. Three films are reviewed including *Pulmonary Selfcare,* produced by Encyclopaedia Britannica, *PEP Series,* produced by the Georgia Lung Association, and *I Am Joe's Lung,* distributed by Pyramid Films.

Also included is a list of educational pamphlets, brochures, and the addresses of organizations that have additional information regarding pulmonary rehabilitation and home care relative to their disciplines.

Audiovisual Aids

Pulmonary Selfcare: A Program for Patients, * by consultants Linda Doyle, R.N., M.N.C.; Eileen Hagarty, R.N., M.S.; John E. Hodgkin, M.D.; Leonard D. Hudson, M.D.; Karen Schaffran Larson, R.R.T., Marion T. Leone, R.N.; William Walthall, R.P.T., B.S.; and Wileen G. Zorn, R.N., M.S. Four videocassette tapes, 3/4" u-matic, 1/2" Beta, 1/2" VHS. Chicago: Encyclopaedia Britannica Educational Corporation, 1980. $995 (complete set of 4 videocassettes).

Pulmonary Selfcare: A Program for Patients is just that—a series of videocassettes that teach obstructive COLD patients how to manage their breathing problems in the home and work environment. The four videocassette tapes attempt to teach patients in simple terminology and in real, uncontrived, at-home settings the technical skills of caring for their pulmonary problems. The series uses real patients in their everyday domestic, occupational, and recreational surroundings.

Accompanying the tapes is a 48-page manual for patients and their families, which contains basic information written in lay language about how the respiratory system functions. The manual has very clear and easy-to-see line illustrations depicting the breathing lessons in the videocassette

---

*From O'Ryan J.A.: Film review. *Respir. Care* 28:96–98, 1983. Used by permission.

234

series. Two large posters are included that illustrate some basic warm-up exercises and bronchial drainage positions. The manual follows the video-cassette series in chronological order; however, the manual is written and illustrated well enough that it can be used independently or as a take-home manual for the patient. The manuals are $2.50 each if 40 or fewer are ordered; the price is reduced to $2.25 if more than 40 are ordered.

An instructor's guide is also included with the series. The 16-page pamphlet merely describes the tape series and gives a few general teaching principles and hints on how to use the tapes to the fullest benefit for the patient. Some additional resources are listed at the back. The manual sells for $1.00.

Collectively, the series is designed to teach the patient the basic facets of living and coping with COLD. Each tape stands on its own merits, however, and does not rely on a successive tape in the series to complete a particular breathing lesson or concept of self-care. This means that a patient could watch one tape per visit, practice what is viewed on the tape at home, and see the next tape on another visit. Each tape runs an average of only 24 minutes, minimizing the chance of viewer boredom or lack of attention. The pace of each tape allows the viewer to observe the demonstration of a particular breathing technique, try the technique briefly himself, and then continue viewing without missing any material depicted. In fact, the combination of the pacing and the narrator's soothing "you-can-do-it" tone acts as a reassurance throughout the series.

Videocassette 1, "Living with a Breathing Problem," documents the daily lives of four patients who are learning to cope with their newly diagnosed lung disease. As stated previously, these are real patients, and the viewer is allowed intimate glimpses into their daily lives. The four patients, representing an eclectic population (housewife, journeyman carpenter, small-business owner, and retired marine), all give honest, descriptive accounts of their subjective feelings about their lung disease. The other three tapes show real patients, also. Thus, the viewer can easily find a patient with whom he can identify.

Videocassette 2, "Learning to Breathe Better," is a skill tape that shows the techniques of diaphragmatic/pursed-lip breathing and how to attain total body relaxation for better breathing control. Good animation, coupled with the videocassette patient's performing the same movement, allows the viewer to give an almost simultaneous demonstration. This videocassette also provides a brief review of the procedures at the end of each segment and then a summary at the end of the whole tape. On a negative note, I did notice that the audio portion of pursed-lip breathing was slightly out of sync with the video portion. This may have been a mechanical problem or the result of poor editing, and it was only a minor distraction.

Videocassette 3, "Clearing Your Airways," is devoted exclusively to teaching the patient the basics of proper, controlled coughing techniques, postural drainage, percussions, and vibration. Perhaps the most technical tape of the series, videocassette 3 serves the intended audience well, and very clearly depicts, by a very good combination of animation and actual demonstration, the various airway-clearing techniques. As with videocassette 2, the viewer again is able to participate because of the slower pacing of the tape at crucial parts.

Videocassette 4, "Building Your Strength and Endurance," takes a practical point of view in teaching the patient how to plan daily activities in such a way as to avoid undue shortness of breath and fatigue. Low-level exercises are demonstrated (e.g., arm and leg lifts, walking, and stationary cycling). Pragmatic examples such as the use of cans of food for weights during arm lifts show this tape's ability to focus on domestic resourcefulness.

Videocassette 4 also offers a short but frank discussion on the issue of lovemaking, COLD patients, and their mates. The tape approaches the subject in a sensitive, unembarrassed manner, pointing out that patients should openly express feelings and concerns about sexual preferences to their mates. As with the other tapes, the viewer is encouraged to participate simultaneously; however, the sequences here appear to move a little too fast for comfortable, beneficial participation that would allow quality feedback. Also, diet is given only a brief acknowledgment. I would suggest that a fifth tape be added to cover this subject.

In summary, the filmmakers did what they proposed to do: teach the basic principles of self care to COLD patients. The teaching level of the series is similar to that of a standard daily newspaper—sixth to eighth grade. This would be the correct level to reach the majority of COLD patients.

The videocassettes are well made, and because of their use of real patients, they have that all-important quality of "presence." The series avoids resorting to Hollywood slickness and has a mature, positive, upbeat feel to it. Perhaps most importantly, the tapes avoid depicting stereotypic (i.e., old and crotchety) COLD patients. Indeed, the patients represented appear to be in the age range of the early 40s to mid 60s.

There is one gross omission in this series: none of the patients are shown using oxygen. This omission does tend to minimize the applicability of the scenarios to oxygen-using patients.

While the series is not intended to totally replace one-on-one pulmonary rehabilitation efforts, it does serve as an excellent augmentation to the practitioner's efforts to teach and reinforce proper pulmonary hygiene and breathing control. Perhaps the best critique is one that a viewer would offer: "I have been using the series for approximately 2 years in our out-patient clinic and at bedside. My patients tell me that they approve of it, and I see their approval transformed into action when they are that much more successful in their rehabilitative efforts."

*PEP Series** (Pulmonary Education Package), by Georgia Lung Association consultants Jane G. Gaston; Robert J. DiBenedetto, M.D.; Richard DeBorde, R.R.T., P.A., Steve Hammons, R.R.T., P.A. Ten programs available in videocassettes or slide/tape series. Hilton Head Island, SC: Tri-Comm Productions, Incorporated, 1976. $600 (10 videocassettes), $350 (slide/tape series).

The *PEP Series* is an audiovisual program designed to teach COLD patients and their families about their disease and how to better care for themselves in their home environment.

The brochure published by the Georgia Lung Association to promote the series states that an instructional guide will be provided with suggestions on the usage of the PEP series, along with review booklets of each program for patient use. Neither of these accompanied the set reviewed; therefore, evaluation of them was not possible. In addition, there is a nonrefundable $10 preview charge for each tape. However, if a single program or the series is purchased, this charge will be deducted from the total purchase price.

Each of the 10 tapes could be used individually, or in any combination desired to provide specific education. The topics include the following:

1. How The Lungs Work
2. What Is COPD?
3. Chronic Bronchitis
4. What Is Emphysema?
5. Understanding Asthma
6. Drug Therapy of COPD
7. Inhalation Therapy
8. Oxygen Therapy In The Home
9. Breathing Exercises
10. General Health Measures

The information presented in each tape is generally correct and would be easily understood by patients with a sixth-grade education or better. Cartoon-type drawings represent the characters in each tape, and many of the ideas are presented in a whimsical and amusing manner. Even the diseases are drawn as cartoon characters; however, they are portrayed by very ugly (literally) characters, which may accentuate the patient's attitude who already has a negative outlook on his disease. The illustrations of each dis-

*This section was prepared by Karla Snavely, R.R.T., Pulmonary Rehabilitation Coordinator, Southview Hospital and Family Health Center, Dayton, Ohio.

ease process are well drawn, and the implied anatomy and physiology is easy to visualize.

Each tape provides a review of the preceding information at the end of the program. The tapes also stress following physician's orders and encourage the patient to seek additional information from the physician. However, no suggestion is made that information may be sought from other health professionals, such as respiratory therapists and nurses, who are involved in primary care for COLD patients.

Two of the tapes are somewhat outdated. "Drug Therapy of COPD" does not mention any of the newer bronchodilators, such as Alupent and Theo-Dur. "Oxygen Therapy In The Home" depicts only gaseous oxygen, although liquid systems and oxygen concentrators are now widely used. There is the possibility that the animation used in this tape series may not allow transition of learning to real-life situations.

I Am Joe's Lung* by National Film Board of Canada, available in videocassette. Distributed by Pyramid Films. $425.

I Am Joe's Lung, narrated by Richard Basehart (who also is the voice of the lung) follows "Joe" through his initial episode of severe dyspnea and subsequent hospitalization. A patient viewing the tape could easily identify with "Joe," because the rationalization used by COLD patients to explain their increasing dyspnea is given as background information in Joe's case. Scenes are depicted of the usual testing processes, including pulmonary functions, x-ray, sputum induction, and blood sampling. "Joe's" concern and uncertainty regarding his health is made apparent.

The anatomy and physiology of the pulmonary system is described with excellent use of anatomic models and animation. Asthma, emphysema, and chronic bronchitis are described very well, as are their effects and symptoms. Included is an explanation of the natural defense system of the lung. The O_2/CO_2 transport system is also illustrated.

The necessity of quitting smoking is stressed, and a link between smoking, COLD, and lung cancer is made. Good health care is emphasized in this film along with the primary subject matter, "Joe's" lung.

Pamphlets and Brochures

American Lung Association (or local affiliate)
1740 Broadway
New York, NY 10019

Numerous publications concerning COLD and pulmonary health are available, most are at no charge.

---

*This section was prepared by Karla L. Snavely, R.R.T., Pulmonary Rehabilitation Coordinator, Southview Hospital and Family Health Center, Dayton, Ohio.

Boehringer Ingelheim Ltd.
Ridgefield, CT 06877

"Save Your Breath," by Thomas L. Petty, M.D, gives advice and information about COLD to patients and their families. Cost is $125 for 100 booklets.

Georgia Lung Association, Inc.
1383 Spring Street, N.W.
Atlanta, GA 30309

"Breathing For People With Chronic Lung Disease" gives instruction on pursed-lip breathing, anatomy of the lung, postural drainage, and breathing exercises as well as nutrition and medications. Cost is as follows: 1 to 10 booklets, $2.00 each; 11 to 99 booklets, $1.75 each; 100 books or over, $1.50 each.

Office of Cancer Communications
National Cancer Institute
Building 31, Rm. 10A29
Bethesda, MD 20205

"Clearing The Air" and "Calling It Quits" are two booklets designed as aids to quitting smoking. They present helpful hints about how to quit and how to maintain one's nonsmoking status. The booklets are free.

Organizations*

American Association of Occupational Therapists
1383 Piccard Dr.
Rockville, MD 20850

American Association for Respiratory Therapy
1720 Regal Row
Dallas, TX 75235

American Cancer Society
New York City Division, Inc.
19 W. 56th St.
New York, NY 10019

---

*This section was prepared by Karla L. Snavely, R.R.T., Pulmonary Rehabilitation Coordinator, Southview Hospital and Family Health Center, Dayton, Ohio.

American Dietetic Association
430 N. Michigan Ave.
Chicago, IL 60611

American Heart Association
7320 Greenville Ave.
Dallas, TX 75231

American Lung Association
1740 Broadway
New York, NY 10019

American Medical Association
535 N. Dearborn St.
Chicago, IL 60610

American Nurses Association
10 Columbus Circle
New York, NY 10019

American Osteopathic Association
212 E. Ohio St.
Chicago, IL 60611

American Physical Therapy Association
1156 15th St. N.W.
Washington, DC 20005

Appendix A

Calculating Relative Fractions of Inspired Oxygen (FIo2)*

The following set of equations have been designed to calculate the fraction of inspired oxygen (FI_{O_2}) using a nasal cannula, regardless of the oxygen concentration of the source gas. The parameters required to perform these calculations are tidal volume (VT), respiratory rate (RR), inspiratory-to-expiratory ratio (I:E), flow rate (L/min), inspiratory time (IT), expiratory time (ET), and the oxygen percentage of the source gas (%).

STEP A
Change L/min to cc/sec.
$$\frac{\text{L/min} \times 1{,}000}{60} = A$$

STEP B
Calculate the volume of source gas inspired during the inspiratory time.
$$A \times IT = B$$

STEP C
Calculate the volume of source gas inspired from the anatomic reservoir.
$$(0.25 \times ET) \times A = C$$

STEP D
Calculate the volume of oxygen in the source gas portion of the VT.
$$(B + C) \times (O_2\% \div 100) = D$$

STEP E
Calculate the volume of oxygen in the room air portion of the VT.
$$[VT - (B + C)] \times 0.21 = E$$

STEP F
Calculate the FI_{O_2}.
$$\frac{(D + E)}{VT} = FI_{O_2}$$

---

*Equation was compiled by David Wildasin, R.R.T., Grandview Hospital, Dayton, Ohio.

Sample Problem

Given: VT   500 cc   Calculated: inspiratory time (IT) 1 sec
      RR   20/min   expiratory time (ET) 2 sec
      I:E   1:2
Flow rate   3 L/min
  $O_2\%$ of   92%
source gas

To calculate the IT, divide the RR into 60 (60 ÷ 20 = 3). This determines the total time alotted for the respiratory cycle (3 sec). Divide this by the sum of the I:E ratio (3 ÷ 3 = 1), which determines IT (1 sec). Because the I:E ratio is 1:2, we know that the ET is twice as long as the IT (or 2 sec).

STEP A

$$\frac{3 \times 1000}{60} = 50$$

STEP B

50 × 1 = 50

STEP C

(0.25 × 2) × 50 =
       (0.5) × 50 = 25

STEP D

(50 + 25) × (92 ÷ 100) =
       (75) × (.92) = 69

STEP E

[500 − (50 + 25)] × 0.21 =
      (500 − 75) × 0.21 =
         (425) × 0.21 = 89

Appendix B

High-Calorie, High-Protein Sample Menu*

BREAKFAST
½ cup fruit juice
¾ cup dry cereal
1 slice toast†
½ cup whole milk
½ cup eggnog
1 tsp margarine
coffee or tea†

MIDMORNING SNACK
2 tbsp peanut butter
2 graham cracker squares
½ cup juice

LUNCH
Ham and cheese sandwich:
   2 oz ham
   1 oz cheese
   2 slices bread
   1 tsp mayonnaise
lettuce/tomatoes/Italian dressing
½ cup fruit cocktail
coffee or tea†

MIDAFTERNOON SNACK
Special milkshake:
   ¾ cup ice cream
   ½ cup whole milk
   4 tbsp nonfat dry milk
   1 pkg instant hot cocoa

SUPPER
3 oz baked chicken
1 baked potato
½ cup carrots
1 dinner roll
3 tsp margarine
2 peach halves
coffee or tea†

EVENING SNACK
2 oz cheese, 6 crackers

---

*Menu and diet information were prepared by Rebecca Barnett, R.D., Holly Channell, R.D., Pamela Cleveland, R.D., and Kitty McHugh, R.D., Grandview Hospital, Dayton, Ohio.
†Three tsp of sugar, jelly, or other sources of sugars may be used.

The diet as listed in the meal contains the following approximations:

Calories: 2,800
Carbohydrate 295
Protein 105
Fat 135

If weight loss is indicated, the following sample menu would be more appropriate:
High-Protein, Weight-Reduction Sample Menu

BREAKFAST
½ cup fruit juice
1 slice toast or ¾ cup cereal
½ cup 2% milk
1 tsp margarine
coffee or tea

MIDMORNING SNACK
½ cup 2% milk
1 graham cracker square

LUNCH
2 oz ham
2 slices bread
lettuce with sliced tomatoes
1 tbsp French or Italian dressing
½ cup unsweetened fruit cocktail
1 tsp margarine
coffee or tea

MIDAFTERNOON SNACK
2 oz cheddar or American cheese
6 saltines

SUPPER
2 oz baked chicken (skinned)
1 small baked potato
½ cup carrots
1 tsp margarine
2 unsweetened peach halves
½ cup 2% milk

EVENING SNACK
½ cup 2% milk
3 vanilla wafers

The diet as listed in the meal plan contains the following approximations:

Calories: 1,500
Carbohydrate 155
Protein 75
Fat 65

Notes

1. Nutrient composition of sample menus is for a 70-kg male and designed to provide approximately 40% of total calories as fat to minimize CO_2 production.

2. Protein supplements such as ProPac, Casec, Pro-mix, or powdered milk can be added to liquids for those individuals who cannot meet their protein needs with their daily food intake.

3. A daily multivitamin not to exceed 100% of Recommended Daily Allowances is indicated for individuals who do not have an adequate intake of the basic four food groups.

Index

A

Abdomen: palpation of, 34, 62
Abscess
  cerebral, 49
  pulmonary, 49
Absolute intravascular pressure, 113
Acidemia, 115
  flapping tremor of hands in, 50
Acidosis, 116–117
Addison's disease, 63
Addresses: of organizations, 239–240
Adenosine monophosphate: cyclic, in
  asthma, 19–20
Adenoviral infections: childhood, 34, 49
Aerobic-type training: for inspiratory
  muscle fatigue, 29
Affective teaching, 174, 177
Airflow decrease: in emphysema, 21–22
Airway
  obstruction in asthma, causes of, 17
  resistance in asthma, 20
Albumin: serum, 140
Alcohol: history of, 48
Allergies, 47
Alveolar oxygen tension: decreased,
  115
Amenorrhea, 49
Aminophylline: in inspiratory muscle
  fatigue, 28
AMP: cyclic, in asthma, 19–20
Amperage requirements: for home-care
  equipment, 219
Amyloidosis, 49
Anaphylaxis: slow-reacting substance of,
  in asthma, 19
Anatomy: pulmonary vascular, 112–114
Anemia, 63
Ankle swelling, 49
Anorexia, 49

Anthropometric measurements, 141
Anxiety, 89–102
  biofeedback for controlling, 98–102
  research study on, 90–98
Apical impulse: of heart, 58
Apnea syndromes: sleep, 50
Appendices, 241–245
Around the Clock With COPD, 157
Arteries: pulmonary artery pressure,
  113
Asbestosis, 33, 48
Aspiration, 49
Asthma, 17-21
  airway obstruction in, causes, 17
  biofeedback in, 86–89
  bradykinin in, 19
  discussion of terminology, 88–89
  FEV_1 in, 86
  gas exchange in, 20
  histamine in, 18–19
  mechanics of ventilation in, 20
  peak flow rate in, 86
  physiologic factors in, summary, 21
  prostaglandins in, 19
  psychosocial factors in, 146–147
  pulmonary function studies in, 36–37
  serotonin in, 19
  SRSA in, 19
Atopic dermatitis, 49, 63
Atropine: in asthma, 20
Audiovisual aids, 234–238
Auscultation, 34, 60–62
  of heart sounds, 62
Autogen HT-1, 91
Autogen HT-2, 91
Autogen 1700, 91, 103
Autogen 3400, 91
Autogenic training, 160
Autonomic dysfunction: in asthmatics,
  20

247

B

Beck depression scale, 90
Behavioral techniques, 160–162
Bennett MA-1 ventilator, 223
Bennett PR-2 ventilator, 223
Berylliosis, 48
Beta adrenergic blockade: in asthma, 20
Bicarbonate, 138
Biofeedback, 82–83, 85–111, 160
  in anxiety control, 98–102
  in asthma, 86–89
  breathing retraining with, 102–109
  Certification Institute of America, 109–110
  in dyspnea control, 98–102
  in emphysema, 88–89
  equipment, 91, 92
  professional qualifications for performing, 109–110
  review of literature, 86–89
  for weaning from respirators, 108–109
Bird Mark 7 ventilator, 223
Blood
  chemistry analysis, 35
  count, 34
    white cell, 35
  gases, arterial, 37
  pressure, and biofeedback, in anxious patients, 94
  urea nitrogen, 143
Bradykinin: in asthma, 19
Breath
  shortness of
    degree of, graded from 0 to 4, 15
    scale for, intensity of, 108
  sounds
    bronchial, 61
    bronchovesicular, 61
Breathing
  cold, dry air, and asthma, 20
  control of
    in bronchitis, chronic, 24
    in emphysema, 23
  diaphragmatic pursed-lip, 66–69
  patterns, 51
  resistance, 104–108
  training
    with biofeedback, 102–109

definition of, 64
  principles of, 64–66
  task-specific, concept of, 65
  techniques, 66–71
  work of, 27–28
    in emphysema, 102
Breathlessness, 49
Brochures, 238–239
Bronchial breath sounds, 61
Bronchial lability index, 43
Bronchiectasis, 34
Bronchitis, chronic, 23–24
  control of breathing in, 24
  discussion of terminology, 88–89
  gas exchange in, 24
  lung volumes in, 23–24
  mechanics of ventilation in, 24
  physiologic factors in, summary, 25
  psychosocial factors in, 148
Bronchoconstriction: exercise-induced, studies to determine, 42–43
Bronchogenic carcinoma, 48
  metastatic, 34
Bronchopulmonary segments, 54, 57
Bronchovesicular breath sounds, 61
Buffering capacity: in chronic bronchitis, 24
BUN, 143

C

Calcium: dietary, 144
Caloric requirements: relation to oxygen requirements, 136–137
Cancer
  (See also Carcinoma)
  psychosocial factors in, 148
  self-help groups, 155
Cannula: nasal, 126–129
Capacity
  functional residual, in emphysema, 21
  total lung (see Total lung capacity)
  vital (see Vital capacity)
Carbohydrates, 138, 142
Carbon dioxide
  analysis of expired gas for, 41
  arterial
    in bronchitis, chronic, 24
    in emphysema, 22

elimination, 44
  metabolism and, 138
  retention, 50
  tension, arterial, 8–9
Carbonic acid, 138
Carcinoma
  (*See also* Cancer)
  bronchogenic, 48
    metastatic, 34
Cardinal symptoms, 33, 47
Cardiopulmonary stress testing, 41
Cardiorespiratory insufficiency, 49
Cardiovascular system: review of, 49
Cell-mediated immune responses: and
  malnutrition, 141
Cerebral
  abscess, 49
  hypoxia (*see* Hypoxia, cerebral)
  responses to chronic hypoxemia, 117
Cervical lymphadenopathy, 52
Charting and reporting systems, 191–
  192
  examples
    departmental charting form, 194
    initial assessment report, inpatient,
      193
    initial assessment report,
      outpatient, 195
    reassessment report, outpatient,
      196
Chest
  examination of, 53–62
  palpation of, 57–60
  percussion of, 60
  pigeon, 34
  relaxation, 100–101
  wall, movement of, 58–59
  x-ray, 35
Childhood history, 33, 49
Children
  adenoviral infections in, 34, 49
  asthma in, biofeedback for, 86–89
  measles in, 34, 49
  pertussis in, 49
  sexuality and disability, 165
  teaching, 177
Circulation: pulmonary and systemic,
  pressures in, 114
Circulatory function: effects of training
  on, 11

Ciurass-type ventilators, 223
Climbing stairs, 71, 73, 76–77
  technique for, 76–77
Clubbing, 34, 50, 52–53
  hallmark of, 53
CO_2 (*see* Carbon dioxide)
Coccidioidomycosis, 48
Cognitive teaching, 174, 177
Collateral vessels, 34
Community services: for home
  ventilator care, 229–230
Compliance: definition of, 176
Consultants: home-care, 208–209
Coping: maladaptive, 153
Corticocerebellar degeneration, 34
Cost
  of home care, 206–208
  of home ventilator care, 217–218
  of oxygen
    delivery system, comparisons of,
      124
    transtracheal, 132
  of ventilator, home, 226
Crackles, 61–62
Creatine kinase: during asthma attack,
  26
Creatinine excretion: 24-hour urinary,
  140
Cyanosis, 63
Cycle ergometer, 40, 71, 74, 76, 79
Cyclic adenosine monophosphate: in
  asthma, 19–20
Cycling, 71–72
Cylinder: oxygen, 121–123

                    D

Davis' headband hook, 128
Death
  and dying, patient's rights, 157–159
  medical-legal-ethical definition of,
    158
Decontamination: of home ventilator
  care equipment, 227-229
Departmental charting form: example
  of, 194
Departmental layout, 193, 195–196,
  197
  example of treatment room, 197

Depression, 89, 97–98
  scale, Beck, 90
Dermatitis
  atopic, 49, 63
  protein deficiency causing, 141
Diagnostic techniques: for assessing
    pulmonary dysfunction, 32–45
Diaphragm, fatigue of, 24–27
  central, 25
  EMG testing for, 104–107
  peripheral, 25
Diaphragmatic pursed-lip breathing,
    66–69
Diarrhea: chronic, 49
Diet: sample menus, 243–244
Dietician
  discharge planning duties of, 200
  role in pulmonary rehabilitation, 188
Diffusing capacity, 37
Disability
  sexuality and, 162–165
  socioeconomic factors and, 13, 14
Discharge
  equipment and supply listing for
      home ventilator care, 225
  planning duties of rehabilitation
      team, 200
Driving pressure, 113
Drugs (see Medications)
Dying patient
  home care for, 216
  rights of, 157–159
Dysphagia, 49
Dyspnea, 14
  biofeedback for controlling, 98–102
Dysuria, 49

E

Ear
  oximeter, Hewlett-Packard, 40
  oximetry, 41
Eczema: infantile, 49
Education
  family, checklist for home ventilator
      care, 220–221
  literature, examples of, 185
  pamphlets and brochures, 238–239
  patient, 173–181
    (See also Teaching)

checklist for home ventilator care,
    220–221
  evaluation of, 177–178
  group learning, 177
  motivation to learn, 175–176
  objectives of, 173–175
  objectives of, example, 174
  regarding disease process, 27
Egophony, 61
Elastic recoil: in chronic bronchitis, 23
Elderly
  calcium balance in, 144
  micronutrient deficiency in, 139–140
  nutritional status of, 135
  sexuality in, 165
  vitamin deficiency in, 144
Electrode placement: for EMG
    feedback, 91, 92
Electromyography (see EMG)
Electrophoresis: protein, 35
Embolus: pulmonary, 49
Emerson 3-PV Post-Op ventilator, 223
EMG fatigue testing, 104–107
EMG feedback
  in anxious patients, 94
  from arm, in asthma, 86
  electrode placement for, 91, 92
  in emphysema, 88
  frontalis, in asthma, 86
  intercostal, 96
  pectoral, upper, 97
    chest recording of, 104
Empathy: in teaching-helping
    relationship, 179–180
Emphysema, 21–23
  biofeedback in, 88–89
  control of breathing in, 23
  discussion of terminology, 88–89
  EMG feedback in, 88
  gas exchange in, 22–23
  lung volumes in, 21
  mechanics of ventilation in, 21–22
  physiologic factors in, summary, 23
  relaxation in, 88
  work of breathing in, 102
  x-ray in, chest, 35
Energy stores, 140
Environmental history, 33, 47, 48
Eosinophil count, 35
Epigastric pain: postprandial, 49

Equations: for calculating relative
    fractions of inspired oxygen,
    241–242
Equipment
    biofeedback, 91, 92
    home-care (*see* Home care,
        equipment)
    home ventilator care (*see* Home
        ventilator care, equipment)
    rehabilitation, 192–193
    list of, 197
    supplier, role in home ventilator
        care, 215–216
    testing, 197
Ergometer: cycle, 40, 71, 74, 76, 79
Erythema nodosum, 50, 63
Erythrocytosis, 35
Ethical definition: of death, 158
Examination (*see* Physical examination)
Exercise
    definition of, 64–65
    duration of, 80
    frequency of, 80
    -induced bronchoconstriction, studies
        to determine, 42–43
    intensity of, 78–80
    mode of, 80
    prescription, 78–81
    principles of, 64–66, 71–72
    program, criteria of, 71
    protocols, 37–40
        modified Naughton-type, 38
    range of motion, 69–71
    rehabilitative objectives of, 71
    spring-type, 37
    steady-state, 37, 42
    studies, pulmonary, 37–43
    techniques of, 72–78
    testing
        contraindications to, 38, 39
        indications for, 38, 39
        progressive standardized tests, 40–
            42
        termination, indications for, 38
    tolerance levels, 14–15
Expanded Technologies' Rockwell
    AIM-65, 91
Expiratory
    flow rates, 36
    -inspiratory ratios, 67–68

volume, forced, 36
    in asthma, 86
Eyes: examination of, 52

F

Face: examination of, 51
Family
    education checklist for home
        ventilator care, 220–221
    history, 33, 47, 48
    as primary care givers for home
        ventilator patient, 212, 213,
        216–217
    responsibilities for home care, 201–
        203
Fat(s), 138, 142–143
Fatigue, 50
    diaphragmatic (*see* Diaphragm,
        fatigue of)
    inspiratory muscle, 28–29
Feedback
    biofeedback (*see* Biofeedback)
    bitone derivative, 103
    EMG (*see* EMG feedback)
FEV_1, 36
    in asthma, 86
Fibrosis, 48
Fibrothorax, 49
Finger(s)
    clubbing of, 34, 50, 52–53
        hallmark of, 53
    palpation of, 34
    temperature of, in anxious patients,
        95
FI_{O_2}: calculation of, 241–242
Fissures, 46–47
Fitness, physical, 5, 6–8
    definition of, 6
Forced expiratory volume, 36
    in asthma, 86
Forced vital capacity, 36
Fremitus
    tactile, 59–60
    vocal, 59
Friction rub: pleural, 62
Frontalis electromyography feedback:
    in asthma, 86
Functional residual capacity: in
    emphysema, 21

Funding: of rehabilitation program, 183
Fundoscopic examination, 52

G

Gas
  arterial blood, 37
  exchange
    in asthma, 20
    in bronchitis, chronic, 24
    in emphysema, 22–23
    equations of, 42
Gastroesophageal incompetence, 33
Gastrointestinal diseases, 33
Gastrointestinal system
  protein starvation and, 141
  review of, 49
Genitalia: external, examination of, 62
Genitourinary system: review of, 49
Glycogen, 138
Group learning, 177
Guided imagery, 160, 161
Gums: examination of, 53

H

Halitosis, 53
Hands
  examination of, 52–53
  -on evaluation, 46–63
Head: examination of, 51
Heart
  apical impulse of, 58
  disease, 33
  failure, congestive, 49
  rate, and biofeedback in anxious
    patients, 95
  responses to chronic hypoxemia, 117
  sounds, auscultation of, 62
Heimlich's transtracheal oxygen
    system, 130–132, 133
Hematopoietic system: and protein
    starvation, 141
Hematuria, 49
Hemoglobin, 34
Hewlett-Packard ear oximeter, 40
Histamine: in asthma, 18–19
Histiocytosis X, 63
Histoplasmosis, 48

History, 32–34, 46–49
  childhood, 33, 49
  environmental, 33, 47, 48
  family, 33, 47, 48
  in nutritional assessment, 141
  occupational, 33, 47, 48
  personal, 48
  smoking, 33, 47, 48
  summary of sections of, 50
Home care, 190, 199–210
  consultants, 208–209
  cost of, 206–208
  equipment
    desired operating characteristics
      of, 206
    selection of, 204–205
  family responsibilities, 201–203
  hospital-based, alternative to, 208–
    209
  maintaining therapy standards, 204
  nurse's role in, 200
  oxygen
    delivery systems, 224
    guidelines for prescribing, 123–126
    initial equipment set-up report
      sample, 129
    monthly follow-up report sample,
      130
    vendors, working with, 128–130
  patient responsibilities, 201–203
  quality, assessment of, 205–206
  respiratory therapist's role in, 200
  safe, requirements for, 203–204
  supplier (see Supplier)
  team, role of, 199–201
  ventilator (see Home ventilator care)
  visit report, sample of, 202
Home ventilator care, 211–233
  clinical profile of ideal patient for,
    217
  community services, 229–230
  continuing care, 230–232
  cost considerations, 217–218
  equipment
    amperage requirements for, 219
    ancillary, selection of, 222–223
    decontamination, 227–229
    discharge, listing of, 225
    evaluation of home, 218–220
    follow-up care, 230–232

follow-up form, example of, 231
home-care planner's role in, 215
identifying prime candidate for, 212–213
infection control procedures, 227–229
instructional routine, 220–222
    patient and family education checklist, 220–221
nurse's role in, 215
patient profile types, 212, 213
physician's role in, 214
primary care givers, family as, 212, 213, 216–217
psychological consultant's role in, 214
respiratory therapist's role in, 214–215
social service planner's role in, 215
summary of fundamental assessment criteria needed for successful home care, 214
supply listing, discharge, 225
team members, 213–216
ventilator considerations, 223, 226–227
    backup ventilator, 226–227
    cost, 226
    ease of operation, 226
    power source, 226
    reliability, 226
    safety, 223, 226
    versatility, 226
Hoover's sign, 59
Horner's syndrome, 52
Hospital
    -based home care, alternative to, 208–209
    ventilator care costs, vs. home, 218
Host defense mechanism, 141
Hypercapnia, 24
Hyperinflation: of lungs, 34
Hypertension, 50
    pulmonary, 115–118
    pathophysiology of, 115–117
Hyperthyroidism, 50
Hypertrophic pulmonary osteoarthropathy, 34, 50, 53
Hyperventilation: and asthma, 20
Hypnosis, 160
Hypocarbia, 20

Hypophosphatemia, 27
Hypoxemia
    asthma and, 20
    chronic, organ responses to, 117–118
Hypoxia, 115–116
    alternative mechanisms of action of, 116
    cerebral, chronic
        diaphragmatic pursed-lip breathing and, 66–68
        range of motion exercises and, 69

I

I Am Joe's Lung, 238
I:E ratios, 67–68
Imagery: guided, 160, 161
Immune responses: cell-mediated, and malnutrition, 141
Immunoglobulin
    A, and malnutrition, 141
    levels, 35
Immunologic diseases, 33
IMT, 81–82
    device, illustrations of, 82
Infantile eczema, 49
Infarction: myocardial, 49
Infection, 135–136
    adenoviral, childhood, 34, 49
    control procedures for home ventilator care, 227–229
Initial assessment reports, examples of
    inpatient, 193
    outpatient, 195
Inpatient, 190
    initial assessment report, example of, 193
Inspiratory
    -expiratory ratios, 67–68
    muscle
        fatigue, 28–29
        training, 81–82
        training device, illustration of, 82
Insurance plans: and home-care services, 207
Intercostal EMG feedback, 96
Interstitial diseases: on chest x-ray, 35
Interstitial pneumonitis, 48
Interview: patient, 46–49

Intravascular pressure: absolute, 113
Iron requirements, 136

J

Jugular venous distention, 52

K

Kwashiorkor, 139, 140, 141
Kyphosis, 34

L

Laboratory tests, 34–35
  in nutritional assessment, 141
Lactic acid, 138
Laryngeal obstruction, 53
Learning
  (See also Education, patient; and
    Teaching)
  group, 177
Legal definition: of death, 158
Legislators: and cost of home care, 208
Life Products LP-4 ventilator, 223
Liquid oxygen, 121–123
Listener: in teaching-helping
    relationship, 179
Literature, 238–239
  on biofeedback, review of, 86–89
  marketing/educational, examples of,
    185
  on quality of life, review of, 151–152
Liver: low-lying, 34
Living will, 158
Lobes: movement of, 59
Locomotor systems: review of, 50
Lordosis, 34
LP-4 ventilator, 223
Lung
  (See also Pulmonary)
  anatomy of, 18
  cancer (see Cancer)
  capacity, total (see Total lung
    capacity)
  disease, pathophysiology of, 17–31
  hyperinflation of, 34
  I Am Joe's Lung, 238
  surface markings (see Surface
    markings of lungs)

  volumes
    in bronchitis, chronic, 23–24
    determinations of, 37
    in emphysema, 21
Lymphadenopathy: cervical, 52
Lymphocyte count, 141

M

Maladaptive coping, 153
Malaise: general, 50
Malnutrition
  causes of, 135
  protein calorie, 136
  types of, 140
Marasmic protein deficiency, 139, 140,
    141
Marketing of pulmonary rehabilitation
    program, 182–185
  announcement to market, example
    of, 184
  literature, examples of, 185
Measles: childhood, 34, 49
Mediastinum, 57
Medical definition: of death, 158
Medical illnesses: past, 49
Medications, 50
  in inspiratory muscle fatigue, 28
  oxygen and, transtracheal, 132
Meditation, 160
Menus: sample, 243–244
Mesothelioma, 48
Metabolic changes, 135–136
Metabolic system: review of, 50
Metastatic bronchogenic carcinoma, 34
Micronutrients, 143–144
  deficiency, in elderly, 139–140
Miliary tuberculosis, 52
Mineral
  requirements, 136
  supplements, 144
Mononeuropathy, 34
Motion: range of motion exercises,
    69–71
Motivation: to learn, 175–176
Mouth: examination of, 53
Movement therapy, 160
Multidisciplinary rehabilitation team,
    153–155, 185–189
  dietician (see Dietician)

discharge planning duties of, 200
in home care, 199–201
in home ventilator care, 213–216
  follow-up and continuing care
    duties, 230–232
members, roles of, 186–189
nurse (*see* Nurse)
occupational therapist (*see*
    Occupational therapist)
pastoral care (*see* Pastoral care)
physical therapist (*see* Physical
    therapist)
physician (*see* Physician)
professional qualifications for
    performing biofeedback,
    109–110
psychiatrist (*see* Psychiatrist)
psychologist (*see* Psychologist)
respiratory therapist (*see* Respiratory,
    therapist)
social worker (*see* Social worker)
Muscle
  fiber types, properties of, 26
  inspiratory (*see* Inspiratory, muscle)
  pectoral (*see* Pectoral muscle)
  relaxation, 85
  somatic, stores, 140
  training, in inspiratory muscle
    fatigue, 28–29
Myocardial infarction, 49
Myopathy, 50

N

Nasal
  cannula, 126–129
  passages, patency of, 53
  polyps, 53
Naughton-type exercise protocol:
    modified, 38
Neck
  examination of, 52
  palpation of, 34
Nervous system: review of, 49
Neuropsychologic effects: of oxygen
    therapy, 149
Nitrogen
  balance, 143
  blood urea, 143
  urinary urea, 143

Nocturnal Oxygen Therapy Trial, 119
Nonphysiologic factors, 13–14
NOTT (Nocturnal Oxygen Therapy
    Trial), 119
Nurse
  discharge planning duties of, 200
  home-care functions of, 200
  role in home ventilator care, 215
  role in pulmonary rehabilitation, 187
Nutrition, 135–145, 243–245
  assessment, 140–141
    initial, 141
  diaphragm muscle mass and, 26
  sample menus, 243–244
  therapy, 141–144

O

O$_2$ (*see* Oxygen)
Objective gains, 5, 8–10
Objectives
  of oxygen therapy, 119–121
  of patient education, 173–175
    example of, 174
  of pulmonary rehabilitation program,
    6–7
Observation, 34, 51
Occupational history, 33, 47, 48
Occupational therapist, 65
  discharge planning duties of, 200
  role in pulmonary rehabilitation,
    187–188
Organ responses: to chronic
    hypoxemia, 117–118
Organizations
  addresses of, 239–240
  self-help groups, 155–157
Orthopnea, 49
Osteoarthropathy: hypertrophic
    pulmonary, 34, 50, 53
Outpatient, 190
  initial assessment report, example of,
    195
  reassessment report, examples of,
    196
Oximeter: Hewlett-Packard ear, 40
Oximetry: ear, 41
Oxygen
  analysis of expired gas for, 41
  concentrator, 121–123

Oxygen *(cont.)*
  cylinder, 121–123
  delivery systems, 121–132
    benefits of, 125
    considerations, 121
    cost comparisons, 124
    future techniques, 133
    limitations of, 125
  home-care *(see* Home-care, oxygen)
  inspired, calculating relative fractions
    of, 241–242
  liquid, 121–123
  requirements, relation to caloric
    requirements, 136–137
  supplemental, and exercise, 80–81
  supplier, responsibilities of, 123
  tension, alveolar, decreased, 115
  tension, arterial, 8–9
    decreased, 115
    in emphysema, 22
  therapy, 112–134
    neuropsychologic effects of, 149
    Nocturnal Oxygen Therapy Trial, 119
    objectives of, 119–121
    patient selection for, 118–119
  transport, 44
  transtracheal, 130–132, 133
  uptake, maximal, 7–8

P

Pa_{CO_2}, 8–9
Pain: postprandial epigastric, 49
Palpation, 34
  of chest, 57–60
  of neck, 52
Pamphlets, 238–239
Pancoast's tumor, 52
Panic training, 27
Pa_{O_2} *(see* Oxygen, tension, arterial)
Passive will: and biofeedback, 99–100
Past medical illnesses, 49
Past surgical illnesses, 49
Pastoral care member
  discharge planning duties of, 200
  role in pulmonary rehabilitation, 188–189
Pathophysiology: of lung disease, 17–31

Patient
  education *(see* Education, patient)
  interview, 46–49
  responsibilities for home care, 201–203
  rights, death and dying, 157–159
Peak flow rate: in asthma, 86
Pectoral muscle, upper
  EMG feedback, 97
  chest recording of, 104
  relaxation, 100–101
Pectoriloquy, 61
Pectus excavatum, 34
PEFR: in asthma, 86
PEP Series (Pulmonary Education Package), 237–238
Peptic ulcer, 49
Percussion: of chest, 60
Personal history, 48
Personnel
  (See also Multidisciplinary rehabilitation team)
  obtaining, 189–190
Persuasion: definition of, 176
Pertussis: childhood, 49
Phase I-IV concept, 191
Physical examination, 34, 50–63
  in nutritional assessment, 141
  summary of sections of, 63
Physical fitness, 5, 6–8
  definition of, 6
Physical therapist
  discharge planning duties of, 200
  role in pulmonary rehabilitation, 187
Physical therapy, 160
Physical training
  effects on circulatory and respiratory function, 11
  program, objectives and benefits of, 10
Physician, role of
  in discharge planning, 200
  in home ventilator care, 214
  in prescribing oxygen, 123
  in rehabilitation, 186
  in selection of home-care equipment, 204–205
Physiologic factors, 14–15
  in asthma, summary of, 21

in bronchitis, chronic, summary of, 25
in emphysema, summary of, 23
Physiologic function: of pulmonary vascular bed, 112–114
Physiologic picture, 43–44
Pigeon chest, 34
Pleural friction rub, 62
Pneumonitis: interstitial, 48
Polyneuropathy, 34
Polyps: nasal, 53
Postprandial epigastric pain, 49
Power source: for home ventilator, 226
Presenting complaints, 33, 47
Pressure
    absolute intravascular, 113
    blood, and biofeedback, in anxious patients, 94
    driving, 113
    pulmonary artery, 113
    in pulmonary circulation, 114
    pulmonary vascular, 113
    in systemic circulation, 114
    transmural, 113
Print media, 238–239
Professional qualifications: for performing biofeedback, 109–110
Profile of Mood States, 90
Prostaglandins: in asthma, 19
Prostate gland: examination of, 62
Protein
    calorie malnutrition, 136
    depletion, 139, 140, 141
    electrophoresis, 35
    requirements, 143
    starvation, 141
    stores, visceral, 140
Psychiatrist
    discharge planning duties of, 200
    role in pulmonary rehabilitation, 189
Psychologist
    discharge planning duties of, 200
    role in home ventilator care, 214
    role in pulmonary rehabilitation, 189
Psychomotor teaching, 174, 177
Psychosocial factors, 13–14, 65–66, 146–172
    in asthma, 146–147

in bronchitis, chronic, 148
in cancer, 148
death and dying, patient rights relating to, 157–159
self-help groups, 155–157
sexuality and disability, 162–165
treatment of whole person, 159–160
Publications (see Literature)
Pulmonary
    (See also Lung)
    abscesses, 49
    artery pressure, 113
    cardiopulmonary stress testing, 41
    circulation, pressures in, 114
    dysfunction, diagnostic techniques for assessing, 32–45
    embolus, 49
    exercise studies, 37–43
    function studies, 36–37
    hypertension, 115–118
        pathophysiology of, 115–117
    osteoarthropathy, hypertrophic, 34, 50, 53
    rehabilitation (see below)
    responses to chronic hypoxemia, 117
    vascular
        anatomy, normal, 112–114
        physiology, 112–114
        pressures, 113
Pulmonary rehabilitation
    candidate, selection of, 5–16
    equipment, 192–193
    list of, 197
    paradigm of, 153
    performance of, where and when, 190–191
    phase I-IV concept, 191
    program
        flow plan for, 182, 183
        marketing of (see Marketing)
        objectives of, 6–7
        obtaining personnel for, 189–190
        starting of, 182–198
        starting of, table relating to, 198
    team (see Multidisciplinary rehabilitation team)
    techniques, 64–84
Pulmonary Selfcare: A Program for Patients, 234–237

Q

Quality of life, 159
  components of, 151
  review of literature, 151–152

R

Range of motion exercises, 69–71
Rectum: examination of, 62
Referrals, 183–184
Registered nurse (*see* Nurse)
Rehabilitation
  definition of, 173
  pulmonary (*see* Pulmonary
    rehabilitation)
Relaxation, 27
  in asthma, 86–88
  chest, 100–101
  in emphysema, 88
  muscle, 85
  pectoral, upper, 100–101
  progressive, 160, 162
  tapes, 100
Renal function: in chronic hypoxemia,
    117–118
Reporting systems (*see* Charting and
    reporting systems)
Residual capacity: functional, in
    emphysema, 21
Residual volume
  in asthma, 20
  in bronchitis, chronic, 24
  in emphysema, 21
Resistance breathing, 104–108
Respirator (*see* Ventilator)
Respiratory
  cardiorespiratory insufficiency, 49
  Consultants of Dayton, 209
  distress, 51
  function
    effects of training on, 11
    tests, criteria for, 11
    tests, rating of, 12
  therapist
    discharge planning duties of, 200
    home-care functions, 200
    role in home ventilator care,
      214–215
    role in pulmonary rehabilitation,
      186–187

tract, upper
  diseases of, 33
  examination of, 53
Rest: for muscle fatigue, 28
Review of systems, 49–50
Rhinitis: allergic, 49
Rights of patients: related to death and
    dying, 157–159
Rockwell AIM-65: Expanded
    Technologies', 91
Rub: pleural friction, 62

S

Safety, home-care
  requirements for, 203–204
  ventilator, 223, 226
Sarcoidosis, 63
Schistosomiasis, 48
Scoliosis, 34
Self-esteem, 13
Self-help groups, 155–157
Senility
  diaphragmatic pursed-lip breathing
    and, 66–68
  range of motion exercises and, 69
Serotonin: in asthma, 19
Sexuality: and disability, 162–165
Shortness of breath (*see* Breath,
    shortness of)
Skin
  examination of, 63
  fold measurements, triceps, 140
  protein starvation and, 141
  tests in nutritional assessment, 141
Sleep apnea syndromes, 50
Slow-reacting substance of anaphylaxis:
    in asthma, 19
Smoking history, 33, 47, 48
Social worker
  discharge planning duties of, 200
  role in home ventilator care, 215
  role in pulmonary rehabilitation,
    188
Socioeconomic factors, 13, 14
Somatic muscle stores, 140
Sounds
  breath (*see* Breath, sounds)
  heart, auscultation of, 62
Spirometry, 36, 43

Sputum: examination of, 35
SRSA: in asthma, 19
Stair climbing, 71, 73, 76–77
  technique for, 76–77
Stem-cell proliferation: and
  malnutrition, 141
Stress, 89
Subjective feeling scale, 93
Subjective gains, 5, 10–15
Supplier, home-care, 205
  equipment, role in home ventilator
    care, 215–216
  fraud and unethical practices of, 207
  oxygen
    responsibilities of, 123
    working with, 128–130
  role in home ventilator care,
    215–216
Supply listing: discharge, for home
  ventilator care, 225
Surface markings of lungs, 56–57
  anterior aspect, 54
  lateral aspect, 54
  posterior aspect, 54
Surgical illnesses: past, 49
Swimming: aerobic-type, for inspiratory
  muscle fatigue, 29
Symptoms: cardinal, 33, 47
System(s): review of, 49–50
Systemic circulation: pressures in, 114

T

Tactile fremitus, 59–60
Tapes, 234–238
  relaxation, 100
Task-specific breathing retraining:
  concept of, 65
Teaching
  (See also Education)
  affective, 174, 177
  best way of, 176–177
  cognitive, 174, 177
  -helping relationship, 178–180
    empathy in, 179–180
    listener in, 179
  psychomotor, 174, 177
  young learner, 177
Team (see Multidisciplinary
  rehabilitation team)

Teeth: examination of, 53
Temperature: finger, in anxious
  patients, 95
Tension, 89, 97, 98
Testicles: painful, 49
Testing equipment, 197
Therapist
  occupational (see Occupational
    therapist)
  physical (see Physical therapist)
  respiratory (see Respiratory,
    therapist)
Total lung capacity
  in asthma, 20
  in bronchitis, chronic, 23
  in emphysema, 21
Trachea, 57–58
Training
  autogenic, 160
  breathing (see Breathing, training)
  inspiratory muscle, 81–82
    device for, illustration, 82
  muscle, in inspiratory muscle fatigue,
    28–29
  panic, 27
  physical (see Physical training)
Transferrin levels, 140
Transmural pressure, 113
Transtracheal oxygen, 130–132, 133
Treadmill, 40, 71, 72, 74, 76, 78
Treatment room: example of, 197
Tremors, 50
Triceps skin fold measurements, 140
Tuberculosis
  history of, 33
  miliary, 52
Tumor: Pancoast's, 52

U

Ulcer: peptic, 49
Urinary system: review of, 49
Urticaria, 63
UUN, 143

V

Veins: jugular, distention of, 52
Vena caval obstruction: superior, 34
Vendor (see Supplier)

Ventilation
  mechanical (*see* Ventilator)
  mechanics of
    in asthma, 20
    in bronchitis, chronic, 24
    in emphysema, 21–22
Ventilator
  assistance for inspiratory muscle
    fatigue, 28
  flow sheet, 232
  in-home (*see* Home ventilator care)
  weaning from, biofeedback for,
    108–109
Vessels
  cardiovascular system, review of, 49
  collateral, 34
  pulmonary (*see* Pulmonary, vascular)
Visceral protein
  deficiency, 139, 140, 141
  stores, 140
Visual imagery, 160, 161
Vital capacity, 36
  in emphysema, 21
  forced, 36
Vitamin
  deficiency, 144
  requirements, 136
  supplements, 144
VO$_2$ max, 7–8
Vocal cords: examination of, 53
Vocal fremitus, 59
Volume
  forced expiratory, 36
    in asthma, 86
  lung (*see* Lung, volumes)
  residual (*see* Residual volume)

W

Walking, 71, 72
  aerobic-type, for inspiratory muscle
    fatigue, 29
  benefits of, 72–73
  progress sheet, sample of, 75
  techniques of, 72–73, 74
  test, twelve-minute, 40, 73
Weaning: from respirator, biofeedback
  for, 108–109
Weight
  gain, 50
  loss, 50, 135–136
Wheezes, 61
Wheezing, 34
White blood cell count, 35
Whole person: treatment of, 159–160
Will
  living, 158
  passive, and biofeedback, 99–100
Winship's cannula support necklace,
  127
Work of breathing, 27–28
  in emphysema, 102

X

X-rays: chest, 35

Y

Yoga, 160